PENGUIN BOOKS

THE CESAREAN MYTH

Dr. Mortimer G. Rosen is Willard C. Rappleye Professor and Chairman of the Department of Obstetrics and Gynecology at the College of Physicians and Surgeons at Columbia University as well as Director of Obstetrics and Gynecology in the Sloane Hospital for Women of the Presbyterian Hospital of New York City. Born in Brooklyn, Dr. Rosen has held academic positions at the University of Rochester and Case Western Reserve University. He has always practiced medicine as well, specializing in high-risk patients. In the area of research, he pioneered techniques for the study of the fetal encephalogram during labor and fetal behavior states and activity patterns prior to birth. Dr. Rosen has a strong interest in the quality of obstetrical care during pregnancy and labor, and has been active in the debate over the rising cesarean birth rate in the United States. He chaired a National Institutes of Child Health and Human Development panel on cesarean childbirth. Dr. Rosen lives on City Island, New York, with his wife, Dr. Lynn Rosen.

Lillian Thomas is a free-lance writer living in Cambridge, Massachusetts.

THE
CESAREAN
MYTH

**Mortimer Rosen, M.D.,
and Lillian Thomas**

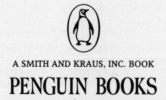

A SMITH AND KRAUS, INC. BOOK
PENGUIN BOOKS

PENGUIN BOOKS

Published by the Penguin Group
Viking Penguin, a division of Penguin Books USA Inc.,
40 West 23rd Street, New York, New York 10010, U.S.A.
Penguin Books Ltd, 27 Wrights Lane,
London W8 5TZ, England
Penguin Books Australia Ltd, Ringwood,
Victoria, Australia
Penguin Books Canada Ltd, 2801 John Street,
Markham, Ontario, Canada L3R 1B4
Penguin Books (N.Z.) Ltd, 182–190 Wairau Road,
Auckland 10, New Zealand

Penguin Books Ltd, Registered Offices:
Harmondsworth, Middlesex, England

First published in simultaneous hardcover and paperback editions
by Viking Penguin, a division of Penguin Books USA Inc. 1989
Published simultaneously in Canada

1 3 5 7 9 10 8 6 4 2

Copyright © Mortimer Rosen and Lillian Thomas, 1989
Illustrations copyright © Viking Penguin,
a division of Penguin Books USA Inc., 1989
All rights reserved

LIBRARY OF CONGRESS CATALOGING-IN-PUBLICATION DATA
Rosen, Mortimer G.
The cesarean myth.
1. Cesarean section—Popular works. I. Thomas,
Lillian. II. Title.
RG761.R73 1989   618.8'6   88-40411
ISBN 0 14 01.1312 6

Printed in the United States of America
Set in Meridien
Designed by Kathryn Parise
Illustrations by Laura Hartman Maestro

For Lynn

CONTENTS

INTRODUCTION

When I began practicing obstetrics in the late 1950s one in every twenty or thirty babies was born by a cesarean delivery. Now more than one in four babies in the United States is born this way. In less than three decades the cesarean birth rate has risen from under 5 percent to 27 percent.

At first the rising rates seemed logical. Cesareans are performed to prevent possible threats to the infant's life or health or to that of the mother. In fact, obstetricians were delivering higher percentages of healthy babies each year. We had begun to develop equipment designed to help us know when there were problems in pregnancy or labor; we had better anesthesia and had developed techniques to make surgery less traumatic. With infant health improving as the number of cesareans increased, it seemed we were doing something right. Like my colleagues, I was performing more cesareans than I had when I started practicing, overseeing difficult vaginal births less often, using the forceps less frequently.

In the mid-1970s, however, the pattern that had been so encouraging changed. We stopped seeing significant improvements in infant mortality and morbidity rates each year. The cesarean birth rate, however, continued to rise, climbing a percentage point or more each year. We were delivering more and more babies by cesarean, but about the same percentage of them died and about the same percentage were born with brain damage or other problems.

The discrepancy between the two rates was apparent by 1979, when the cesarean rate had already reached 16 percent. That year I chaired a National Institutes of Health panel that studied the rising cesarean rate. We concluded that too many cesareans were being done and looked at the individual diagnoses that were resulting in cesareans. In addition, I began to do investigations of my own. I soon came to the firm conclusion that the high cesarean rate was not medically justified. The cesarean had solved some of our problems, but it clearly had failed to solve others. Yet we continued to practice as if it *were* solving those problems. Further, I became convinced that the cesarean birth was not any safer than a vaginal birth for babies in most cases, and that it was much more risky for the mother.

After my experience on the cesarean panel and my early investigations, I began to become concerned. I became more and more aware of the changes that were taking place in medical practice and in people's attitudes toward childbirth.

I specialize in high-risk patients in my practice, women who have had poor pregnancy outcomes in the past or are at risk for poor outcomes. Even with the best, most sophisticated care, we physicians are helpless in certain circumstances. Cerebral palsy and certain other conditions have proved to be intractable problems. We understand them better than we did a few decades ago but often can't prevent them. And despite the belief that a cesarean birth can prevent brain damage, my experience has convinced me that it usually cannot.

I've also become aware of a subtle change in attitudes in court cases in which I am involved as a witness. I have testified as an expert witness in many malpractice cases, and it's become apparent to me that death and damage are no longer viewed simply as tragedies, but as tragic consequences of a mistake made somewhere by someone.

In trying to understand why the cesarean rate continued to climb at such a rapid rate, I began to realize that there was a powerful set of myths associated with cesareans. These myths had grown up quickly over the decades in which cesarean rates rose and are now firmly ensconced. Patients and doctors alike have come to believe that cesareans are as safe as vaginal birth, that they are necessary in a wide range of cases, and that they guarantee a good outcome. I will discuss these myths in detail in this book, but I want to emphasize here that they are myths that have taken hold both in and outside the medical community.

I think they developed as a result of changing attitudes in both the medical and the lay community. Doctors began to act as if the technology being developed could predict and solve all problems. We were generating false confidence and we were beginning to forget that instruments such as electronic fetal monitors were tools to be used by the doctor, not decision-making machines to replace medical judgment.

The second mistake doctors made was to treat the cesarean as a cure-all. If there was any problem in labor, the cesarean was the automatic answer. Even as we were learning that many problems in babies occur long before labor, doctors acted as if all death and injury occurred during birth and therefore could be eliminated by avoiding vaginal birth. This was—is—nonsense.

We also let simplistic guidelines replace good medical judgment. We were learning that many women who had had a cesarean could deliver subsequent babies vaginally, but we continued to follow the outdated prescription, "Once a cesarean, always a cesarean."

On the patient side, there was the development of the expectation of a perfect outcome. Women seem to come in believing that all babies can be born healthy. A dead or damaged baby is no longer simply a tragedy, but an outcome that is someone's fault. People don't seem to think there are things that can go wrong that are simply out of the doctor's control. Perhaps this attitude developed partly because we in the medical community sold our technology and the successes we had too well. Perhaps it is just part of a wider societal shift in attitude. At any rate, the mixture of these changing attitudes was bound to produce more cesareans. Patients expected a good outcome; both patient and doctor believed the cesarean was some sort of guarantee of this; even the doctor who doubted the cesarean was going to make a difference knew that he might be asked in court why he hadn't done everything in his power—i.e., a cesarean—to save the baby. Given the cesarean myths, the explosion in cesarean rates was inevitable. The myths continue to feed the growth in cesarean rates and are always on a collision course with the real world, where babies die and no medical miracle can save them.

Even as I became convinced that the rising rates were a bad trend, I was aware of the difficulty of the issue. No obstetrician can fail to be. I've seen cases where a cesarean could have saved an infant's life: The first breech delivery in which I was involved was a vaginal birth, and the baby died. But I've also seen cases where an unnecessary cesarean had disastrous results. I've seen colleagues sued for failing to perform a cesarean, and I know several who've quit practicing because of a lawsuit or the fear of one. I've seen very difficult vaginal births in which I wondered from beginning to end if I was doing the right thing.

In the end, we must make decisions on the basis of the medical information we have available and the circumstances of a particular case—not on personal fears. We cannot let ourselves practice "defensive medicine," performing procedures to protect ourselves rather than our patients. I remain convinced that too many cesareans are being done and that we must do something to stop the escalating rates. We must put an end to the vicious cycle of misconceptions, unreasonable expectations, and inevitable failures to meet the expectations that have continued to feed the trend. I want to encourage both doctors and patients to break this cycle. In lectures I tell my colleagues, "Look at the statistics, use good medical judgment, don't resort to the cesarean when it's not medically warranted." But I know a doctor who uses good judgment can end up with a bad result. Patients can help break the cycle by being informed, by understanding that there is a certain small risk to any birth. I am convinced that a strong physician-patient relationship is the key both to fulfilling birth experiences for individual women and to reducing the cesarean rate. Choosing an obstetrician with whom she is comfortable is one of the most important things an expectant mother can do. Doctors who have good relationships with their patients are less likely to turn to the cesarean as a way of protecting themselves. I hope that my chapter on choosing a doctor will help women find obstetricians with whom they can establish good relationships. I want doctors and patients alike to realize that the high cesarean rate is unhealthy for everyone, and that by working together they can do something about the problem. That is what I hope this book accomplishes.

THE
CESAREAN
MYTH

1
THE CESAREAN MYTHS

A CESAREAN BIRTH

Mary Elizabeth Clinton arrives at the hospital a little after 3:30 A.M. on June 24. Her husband, Dan, explains to the people at the admitting desk that she's just gone into labor but that she was scheduled for a cesarean in four days. Mrs. Clinton is a little tense. Her due date isn't until July 2; how could her doctor be so far off? She doesn't want to go through what she went through with her son—twenty hours of labor, people poking at her, talking to her, telling her to keep working. She had been scared, tired, and in pain. It was a relief when the doctor finally said the baby wouldn't fit and he was going to do a cesarean. The memory of that long, painful labor hadn't faded much over time. This time, she'd told her friends, at least she wouldn't have to go through that again. Once a cesarean, always a cesarean.

When a resident, Dr. Joe Paterno, comes in to examine her, practically the first thing he says is that many women who've had previous cesareans can deliver subsequent babies normally and that the hospital encourages patients to try to deliver vaginally. Mary Elizabeth shakes her head in irritation, looking at this young man who doesn't look old enough to have finished college, let alone medical school. "I want a cesarean. My doctor, Dr. Collins, said I'd have one. I was scheduled for one already. And anyway, I tried last time and the baby didn't fit. I'm too small down there."

"It's not like a key and lock, Mrs. Clinton," says Joe Paterno. "You don't either fit or not fit. It depends on the baby's size and position and a lot of other things."

"I'm not interested in finding out if I fit or don't fit. I just started labor. I want a cesarean." Dr. Paterno finishes the examination and leaves.

He's back around 4:30 to check on her, and he's still trying to talk her out of the cesarean. Mary Elizabeth absolutely refuses. Dan Clinton is down the hall trying to get hold of his wife's doctor, but when Dan comes back he tells the resident to get busy getting ready for the C-section. Paterno leaves and talks to the head resident briefly. When he comes back he tells the Clintons that they'll start prepping Mary Elizabeth for surgery in about a half hour.

At 5:10 someone puts an IV in Mary Elizabeth's hand. Someone else draws blood. At 5:25 they wheel her into the operating room. Someone washes her back and puts a green sheet over her, as in her last delivery.

A man in surgical greens comes into the room. He introduces himself: Dr. Claude Martel, the anesthesiologist. He says he's going to use an epidural anesthetic. "Last time you had a spinal, and I bet you had headaches," he says. Mrs. Clinton nods her head. "You won't get those with this."

Dan comes in with surgical greens on. He says that Dr. Collins isn't on call tonight, so someone else, a Dr. Greenhagen, will do the cesarean. Dr. Collins had explained to the Clintons that he couldn't guarantee he'd be the one to deliver Mary Elizabeth's baby, but she'd still counted on it, since she was having a scheduled cesarean. Now she'd have some strange doctor. . . .

She lies on her side, and Dan holds her while she follows Dr. Martel's instructions to arch her back. First he puts a little needle in, to deaden the area for the bigger one. There's a long silence, and Mary Elizabeth is conscious of several people moving and talking very quietly behind her. She feels pricks and slight sensations as the big needle is moved. She wonders what's taking so long. Finally the anesthesiologist says, "All right, we'll just wait ten minutes to make sure it takes." She sees by a clock on the wall that it's 5:42.

A woman comes to the table and says, "I'm Dr. Holly Greenhagen. I'll be taking care of you, Mrs. Clinton."

At 5:52 Dr. Martel says he's going to pinch her with a pair of forceps. "You shouldn't feel a thing," he says, smiling. Mary Elizabeth flinches and gives a surprised yelp when she feels a sharp pinch.

"I think we should go with a general," someone says.

"They're going to knock me out, Dan? Is that what that means? I won't be able to see the baby when it comes out?"

"I'm afraid so, Mrs. Clinton," says Holly Greenhagen. "And I'm sorry, but I'm going to have to ask your husband to leave." Mary Elizabeth looks at Dan. "She'll be completely under, so you won't be able to help her out," the doctor tells Dan Clinton. "And it's hospital rules."

The nurses turn Mrs. Clinton over on her back and put a pad under her hip. Then they put drapes over her legs. The doctors leave to scrub. They come back and she's pinched with the forceps again. She still feels it. They put a big black mask over her face. The last thing she sees is the back of a nurse leaving the operating room.

In the meantime sodium pentothal has been placed in the IV infusion to put her to sleep and curare to block her muscles so that she will be paralyzed. She won't be able to breathe on her own, so she'll be intubated—a tube will be pushed down her throat into the trachea, near the lungs, so that oxygen can be pumped in and carbon dioxide taken out. As the drugs take hold, Mary Elizabeth Clinton becomes dizzy, sleepy. In seconds it's all black.

6:06: The patient is finally under. A first-year anesthesiology resident puts a hand under her jaw and tips her head back so that he can intubate her. The tube is to be slipped between her vocal cords and down her windpipe. He looks for her vocal cords with an instrument that looks a bit like a metal tongue depressor but has a light on it. However, he can't see the vocal cords.

6:08: Dr. Martel, who's a senior anesthesiology resident, says he'll intubate the patient. He can't see the vocal cords either. It turns out that Mrs. Clinton is one of a certain number of patients whose vocal cords are very difficult to see; putting this tube down is getting to be a problem.

6:09: Martel tries to pass the tube blindly, just pushing it down where he thinks it should go. It won't go. Another resident tries to find the vocal cords and can't.

6:13: The room is jittery. Martel sends for the senior anesthesiologist. The patient is blue. They pull out the tube and give her oxygen with the face mask before they start again.

6:17: The patient's respiratory system is going into spasm. They're getting a little oxygen into her, but not much. This new problem of spasm—similar to, but worse than, a severe asthma attack—makes her lungs wheeze and closes the tube leading to the lungs' air sacs. The doctors are trying to force oxygen, which she desperately needs, into the patient. They fear her brain is becoming as "blue" from the lack of oxygen as are her fingernails.

6:19: Anna Wienowski, the senior anesthesiologist, comes into the operating room. She gets the tube down on her third try.

6:22: Although there's now plenty of oxygen going below Mary Elizabeth's vocal cords, the smaller tubes leading into the lungs are still in spasm; they're not doing a very good job of getting the oxygen into the air sacs, where it can be transferred into her blood.

6:23: While the anesthesiologists have been struggling to put the patient to sleep and get oxygen into her, the obstetrical team has been waiting at the other end of the table to get started. John Gutman, an obstetrical resident, listens to the baby's heartbeat. It's 50—dangerously low. It should be up around 120 to 180 beats a minute. Although the team would prefer to wait until the mother is stabilized, the crisis in the baby's condition makes it necessary to go in. The baby, like the mother, is being deprived of oxygen.

6:24: Within thirty seconds Greenhagen has cut through the skin, the muscle, and the uterus. She brings out the baby, a six-pound, nine-ounce girl. The infant is very depressed—she's limp, not breathing on her own. It turns out the uterus was also in spasm, and there had been what is called an abruption: The placenta had partially detached during the crisis, perhaps as a result of it. This meant the mother and baby were almost cut off from each other. Not only was the mother not getting enough oxygen, but almost none of the little she had was getting to the baby. The little girl is in jeopardy.

6:26: The baby is handed over to a waiting team of pediatricians. The baby's head is extended as her mother's was and a tube inserted. Two doctors from pediatrics and two nurses surround the baby, giving her care. They suction her lungs through the tube, then begin to give her oxygen. They thread a catheter through the umbilical cord and draw blood. They give her fluids she will need to overcome the effects of the lack of oxygen.

Dr. Greenhagen begins sewing up the mother as quickly as she can. Because of the abruption Mary Elizabeth is bleeding heavily. Paterno and another resident work with Greenhagen. At the other end of the table Dr. Martel, Dr. Wienowski, and a couple of nurses are trying to get as much oxygen into the patient as possible. Mary Elizabeth is still blue.

Dan Clinton is outside the room, standing in the hallway because he couldn't keep himself sitting down in the waiting room. He knows only that more and more people are going into the operating room and everybody is moving quickly.

6:29: The baby's heartbeat is up to 100, and she's starting to revive. They are giving her bicarbonate to offset the effects of extreme acidosis, the result of the oxygen deprivation.

Dr. Greenhagen continues to work on Mary Elizabeth. Normally a cesarean can take an hour and a half to two hours; the team is working at a pace that will close her in thirty minutes. With the crisis still going on at the head of the table, the obstetricians want the stress of surgery out of the way.

6:31: The baby's heartbeat is up to 120. The Apgar score is six (out of a possible ten). The oxygen and fluids are beginning to take effect.

6:33: The baby's heartbeat is 130. She's beginning to look pink.

APGAR SCORING SYSTEM*

Sign	Points Awarded		
	0	1	2
heart rate	absent	below 100	above 100
respiratory effort	absent	slow, irregular	good crying
muscle tone	flaccid	some flexion of extremities	active
reflex irritability	no response	grimace	vigorous
color	blue/pale	body pink, extremities blue**	completely pink

*Scores are normally taken at one and five minutes. There is no difference in health between scores of 7, 8, 9, and 10. A low score (6 or less) at one minute is not significant if it rises above 6 at five minutes.

**Almost all babies lose one point for hands and feet blue at one minute after birth.

6:35: The baby begins to move. Her Apgar is up to eight. She's beginning to breathe on her own and resist the tube. Her arms and legs are moving.

6:38: The baby is resisting the tube so well that one of the pediatricians removes it. She's breathing on her own now and seems to be doing well. The pediatric team begins to relax a little—the immediate crisis is over. But the baby could still have problems caused by the oxygen deprivation; it's too early to tell whether she'll be normal.

6:40: A small cart loaded with tubes and bottles is wheeled out of the operating room, surrounded by five doctors and nurses. Dan Clinton runs up and gets a glimpse of a little baby. One of the nurses recognizes him. "We have to take your daughter to intensive care, Mr. Clinton, but we think she'll be all right."

"How's Mary?"

"They're still closing. They had some problems with the anesthesia. I'm not sure exactly . . . they'll let you know," the nurse says, hurrying into the elevator, where the others have wheeled the cart.

6:44: Dr. Greenhagen is about ten minutes from closing, working rapidly but steadily, sewing the fascia, the lining over the muscle. They have to get her closed so the anesthesia team can take care of the other problems.

6:55: Greenhagen finishes the operation.

7:06: Mary Elizabeth Clinton is pink again. They've overcome the muscle spasm. Oxygen is going in as it should. She's still under deep anesthesia, but she's getting oxygen now. Greenhagen pulls back an eyelid to see if the patient's pupils are dilated—which would be a bad sign. Everything seems to be all right; they just have to wait and hope that over the next hour she'll wake up and say, "Where am I?" Dr. Greenhagen goes out to the hall to talk to Dan.

8:33: Mary Elizabeth Clinton finally wakes up, weak and in pain but apparently with no serious problems. Eleven days later, she and her baby are able to go home, both healthy.

* * *

Cases like Mrs. Clinton's are very rare, but they happen. Because cesareans have become so common and are treated so casually by doctors and patients alike, many women don't stop to consider that they are undergoing major surgery when they undergo a cesarean.

CESAREAN VERSUS VAGINAL BIRTHS IN THE UNITED STATES
1987 (estimated)

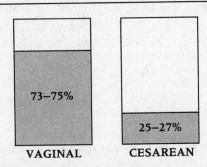

73–75%

25–27%

VAGINAL   **CESAREAN**

[This is an estimate based on figures from 1984, the last year for which firm numbers are available. The source is Shiono, P.H., McNellis, D., and Rhoads, G.G. "Reasons for the Rising Cesarean Delivery Rates 1978–1984." *Obstetrics and Gynecology* 1987, vol. 69, no. 5, p. 696.]

It should be noted that rates for private patients differ from those of nonprivate patients; they are invariably higher. Even in the same hospital, private rates may be 5 to 10 percent higher than rates for nonprivate (clinic) patients.

The number of cesareans performed has increased drastically over the last three decades and particularly in the last fifteen years. In the United States, more than one in four births is a cesarean. Many of those may not be necessary and are often not justified by the medical circumstances. But the continuing growth of the cesarean birth rate has been accepted by the public and the medical community alike. The reason people accept the high rate is that they accept the myths that have grown up concerning the abdominal method of delivering babies.

THE MYTHS

Myth: Cesareans Are Safe

The first of the cesarean myths is the belief that the cesarean is as safe or safer than vaginal delivery. Although cesareans have become far less risky over the years and now pose a very low mortality risk for mothers, they are still a form of major surgery. The fact is that the mother who undergoes a cesarean is at much higher risk of dying than the woman who gives birth vaginally: twice the risk for an elective cesarean; four times the risk for an emergency cesarean. Yet the cesarean has come to be regarded as little different than vaginal birth. In one extreme example of how far this attitude has been taken, the cesarean birth rate for private patients in the practices of many physicians in Brazil is about 90 percent. It is the fashionable way to give birth in Brazil, and women are so convinced the procedure is safe that they elect to have surgery when they have no reason to expect problems in a vaginal delivery.

In addition to the higher mortality rate, the cesarean mother can also take on a whole host of risks that aren't present at all in vaginal births. She will lose at least twice as much blood as a vaginal mother. She may have to receive blood, and there is always a risk of disease or infection from transfusions. Other kinds of infections, related to the surgery itself, may occur in 20 to 40 percent of cesarean patients.

Finally, the cesarean mother will undergo a longer and more painful convalescence. Her average hospital stay will be about twice as long as if she had had a vaginal delivery. She will have pain and may require quite a bit of medication. She may have bad headaches produced by the anesthesia. She may be tired from the loss of blood. At a time she most wants to be with her new baby, she may be in pain or feel extremely sick and tired. The first month of her baby's life is rarely the same as that of a baby born vaginally.

Myth: Cesareans Are Necessary in a Broad Range of Cases

Most women who've had a cesarean believe it was absolutely necessary. Their doctors told them that their babies wouldn't fit or that the infants were at risk or simply that a cesarean was necessary.

The fact is, there is only a small group of situations in which a cesarean is absolutely necessary. These include cases involving certain high-risk patients, some types of breech births, situations in which the placenta is attached in the wrong place, and cases in which there is clear evidence that the infant's health or life is being endangered by vaginal delivery. *Not* included in this category is the repeat cesarean, which accounts for 30 percent of all cesarean births and is a major cause for the rising cesarean birth rate. The belief that all cesarean patients must have subsequent children by the same method is one of the most pervasive and unfounded myths surrounding the cesarean. The decision on whether to perform a cesarean should be made on a case-by-case basis. Decisions are not being made on such a basis, though, because of the belief that cesareans are necessary in all sorts of situations—a slow labor, some slightly abnormal readings on a heart rate monitor, the discovery that the patient is carrying a big baby, and, of course, the fact that the mother has had a previous cesarean.

In recent years, obstetricians have begun to choose a cesarean whenever there is any uncertainty. Thus, although it is possible for most women who've had previous cesareans to deliver vaginally, many doctors routinely stick by the old saying, "Once a cesarean, always a cesarean." And although some types of breech births can be delivered vaginally, most obstetricians call for an operating room as soon as they encounter a breech baby.

We've come to the point that when a doctor finds anything in a pregnancy or labor that is not perfectly normal, a cesarean is likely to be performed. (Doctors do this for a variety of reasons, which I'll discuss later, but essentially they are acting in what they believe to be the best interests of the patients or in what they believe a jury will deem the best interests of the patients, or both.)

This tendency to turn quickly to a cesarean delivery means that cesarean rates will continue to increase, since more women will have a first cesarean, and the vast majority of those will have the operation on subsequent deliveries. We will continue to put more than one of every four mothers at an increased risk to her own health.

Myth: Cesareans Produce
Healthier Babies

What is the reason for putting more mothers at risk? The health of the baby, of course. The cesarean has come to be viewed as a kind of guarantee of a good outcome. Yet the statistics do not indicate an overall improvement in the health of infants with the rise in cesareans (in the areas in which cesareans are genuinely necessary outcomes are better, but the recent dramatic rise in cesareans has not reduced overall infant mortality rates or produced a generation of healthier babies). Although the data indicate that there is no significant difference in the health of babies born vaginally and those delivered by cesarean, there is a belief among many people that if we deliver babies (particularly very premature babies) gently, delicately, like an egg, they'll be okay. They forget that the majority of problems exist before delivery and aren't affected by it: If a baby is missing a finger, delivering that baby by cesarean won't make any difference. And if the baby is already brain damaged, the cesarean birth route will not change that.

The Issues

I don't want to continue to see cases like Mary Elizabeth Clinton's, nor do I want to see more harm come to babies. Nothing is risk free, of course. There will always be tragedies. But I want to keep doctors and patients alike from bringing on needless tragedies and taking needless risks. By explaining what we know about risks in childbirth and by putting to rest the myths about cesareans, I think we can take a big step in that direction. Women who are pregnant should know what is involved in a cesarean, what the risks are, when it is definitely needed, when it may not be necessary. I hope such understanding on the part of patients and some self-examination in the medical community can combine to stop the escalating cesarean rate and the myths that feed that growth. I believe that knowledgeable patients can work with their doctors to lower the cesarean birth rate and still improve the birth rate of healthy babies.

2

UNDERSTANDING THE CESAREAN

HISTORY OF THE CESAREAN

The idea that a child could be born by some other means than a normal birth seems almost magical, and the cesarean has often figured in legend and myth. Hence we have tales of births that were not really births, like the myth of the Greek god Asclepias being cut from his dying mother by his father, Apollo; the legend that Julius Caesar was born by cesarean; or the fate of Shakespeare's Macbeth, who had been promised that "none of woman born" could harm him but died at the hands of Macduff, born by cesarean.

Cesareans actually were performed in ancient times. As long ago as 3,000 B.C. the Egyptians wrote of cesareans, as did ancient Indians, and there is evidence that cesareans were performed by the ancient Greeks, the Romans, the Hebrews, and the Persians. These cesareans weren't miraculous medical events; they were measures of last resort, desperate operations performed on dead or dying women to try to save their infants. Until very recently, obstructed labor (a general term for any labor in which normal birth proves impossible) almost always ended in the death of the mother or the infant, or both. Most cesareans that were performed were postmortem, and the few performed on living women invariably resulted in their deaths. Medical historians doubt that Julius Caesar was actually a cesarean infant because his mother lived for many years after his birth.

Many ancient societies, including Egypt, India, and Rome, had laws regarding postmortem cesareans. In Rome the *Lex caesarea* made it mandatory that in the event of maternal death in advanced pregnancy, the child should be removed from the mother so that even if the child did not survive, it could be buried separately. (The term *cesarean* may come from this law; we know that the term was used by the Romans to refer to the postmortem incision. Other scholars believe it comes from the Latin word *caedere,* to cut.) Later, the early Christian Church was to make similar provisions, in order to save the soul of the child. Priests were instructed in techniques for performing postmortem cesareans.

We have historical records of many postmortem cesareans. In 1317, Robert II of Scotland was delivered by cesarean after his mother fell off her horse and broke her neck. A hunter cut the infant from the dead woman's body. Edward VI of England may have been born by cesarean. His mother, Jane Seymour, died shortly after his birth in 1537.

There are a few records of early cesareans in which the mother survived. Jacob Nufer, a Swiss hog gelder, was said to have delivered his wife's first child by cesarean in the sixteenth century. She reportedly survived to have four more children. If so, she probably was not only the first woman to live through a cesarean, but the first to give birth vaginally following one.

The first successful cesarean in the United States probably took place in the late eighteenth century. The operation remained very rare into the nineteenth century. Physicians developed other means of dealing with obstructed labors, including the use of forceps. They also attempted to induce early labor in some cases to prevent excessive fetal growth. "Fetal destruction," which usually meant dismembering the infant to save the woman's life, appears to have been more common than the cesarean during this time.

More common than any of these alternatives was simple inaction. In 1817 Princess Charlotte of England underwent an obstructed labor. Her physician, Sir Richard Croft, let the labor continue without intervening at all. He could have attempted either a cesarean, which most likely would have resulted in the princess's death, fetal dismemberment of the next king of England, or a forceps birth. Afraid to take any action that might kill a royal family member, Sir Richard did nothing. The infant was stillborn and the princess died. Three months later Sir Richard shot himself. The incident had an impact on medicine—the very gradual shift away from ultraconservatism and nonintervention began around this time.

It was only in the late nineteenth century, with the advent of antiseptic techniques and the use of anesthesia, that the cesarean became an alternative. Gradually doctors learned surgical techniques and were able to counter postoperative infection. They learned where and how to make the incisions. Improvements in operative procedure made all surgery safer, including the cesarean. By the mid-twentieth century, the cesarean had become a standard treatment for obstetrical emergencies. It accounted for about 4 percent of all births. Most doctors still considered it a last resort and were more likely to use forceps in difficult births, but the cesarean was an acceptable procedure.

In the last three decades we have made the cesarean even safer. We have better anesthesia, better operative procedures, better postoperative care. We understand pregnancy and labor better. We have more precise instruments for monitoring pregnancy and labor. The cesarean, for thousands of years tantamount to death for the mother, is now a low-risk procedure.

THE OPERATION—
A BEDSIDE VIEW

The cesarean is an operation, and in many ways it has more in common with other surgical procedures that it does with vaginal delivery. The outcome—the birth of a baby—and many of the emotions of the parents are the same, but the process is very different.

An elective cesarean is the type of procedure typical among women who have had previous cesareans. If the patient or the doctor, or both, does not want to attempt vaginal delivery, or if there is a compelling medical reason not to attempt it, a cesarean is scheduled. It is elective surgery, and like other elective operations, the decision is made in advance, a date set, and plans made ahead of time.

The obstetrician usually tries to set the surgery date around the thirty-ninth week of pregnancy. The object is to perform the cesarean before labor begins, but not before the baby has had the chance to mature. The obstetrician can determine the maturity of the fetus by using ultrasonography or by testing a sample of amniotic fluid. Ultrasound is a noninvasive procedure that allows doctor and patient alike to see an image of the fetus by bouncing sound waves off it and recording their patterns on a screen. Amniocentesis, the process of drawing amniotic fluid from the womb, is a more intrusive procedure that carries some risk and involves inserting a large needle into the woman's abdomen. An ultrasound scan performed before the twentieth week of pregnancy can fairly accurately pin down the date of conception and allow the doctor to predict the woman's due date and schedule the cesarean a few days earlier. If the dates are not certain, it is sometimes necessary to perform amniocentesis just before the surgery to confirm that the infant's lungs are mature enough to function outside the mother.

Until recently most cesarean patients came to the hospital on the night before their surgery. With the trend toward shorter hospital stays in all areas of surgery, it's now common for the patient to arrive the day the cesarean is to be performed. In that case she'll be told not to take any food or fluids after midnight the night before.

In the hospital, a doctor will take a history and give the woman a physical examination. An hour or more before the operation, prepping will begin. The patient's abdomen will be shaved, a urine sample taken. Then an IV will be inserted and blood drawn. The hospital will make sure the blood bank has an adequate supply of the patient's blood type. The patient may get an enema (this varies from doctor to doctor and from hospital to hospital; sometimes the patient is given a choice, sometimes not).

Next nurses will put the woman on a stretcher and wheel her to the operating room. More and more hospitals permit the husband or a companion to go into the operating room with the patient. This person will put on operating room garb.

There is usually a minimum of four medical personnel involved in a cesarean, and often more. The typical cesarean operating staff would include at least one obstetrician, an anesthesiologist, two nurses (one who scrubs and handles instruments, the other a "circulator" who can leave the room to get more staff if necessary), an assistant to the surgeon or, in a teaching hospital, some residents and/or students.

The nurses will next move the patient from the stretcher to the operating table. Above the patient will be a three-and-a-half-foot-diameter light. The nurses cover the woman with sheets and wrap a band around her legs so they won't kick out during the operation. One arm is outstretched, attached to the IV. The other is tightly wrapped to the woman's side (this is to prevent her from reaching for her abdomen during the procedure and also from knocking into the doctors during surgery).

The anesthesiologist now gets to work. Many hospitals ask the husband or companion to leave during the administration of anesthetic. It's a delicate procedure that involves big needles, and many doctors feel it may be unpleasant for the husband and that his reaction can add stress to the anesthesiologist's job. I prefer to have the husband present throughout the procedure.

There are several types of anesthesia. Regional anesthesia deadens just the area affected by the surgery and allows the patient to remain awake during the procedure. General anesthesia puts the woman into a deep, sleeplike state. She will be unconscious during the entire procedure. General anesthesia obviously takes the experience the furthest from a normal birth. The woman and her husband are essentially uninvolved; she is a passive patient being operated on, not the main actor in a process in which the doctor merely assists, as in a vaginal birth. The woman is also passive in a cesarean performed with regional anesthetic, but at least she is aware of the process.

There are two types of regional anesthesia, spinal and epidural. Both are administered with the woman on her side and with her back arched. In the spinal the anesthetic is injected directly into the spinal canal. It paralyzes all the nerves coming from that area of the spinal cord (usually between the third and fourth lumbar vertebrae). The epidural is a more delicate and difficult procedure; it is less risky if done correctly but more difficult to do. It involves paralyzing certain nerves as they emerge from the spinal cord. The anesthesiologist leaves the soft plastic tube in the patient's back after the initial infusion of anesthetic so he or she can continue to put in anesthetic as the procedure progresses.

If the woman gets a general anesthetic, she will receive the sleep-inducing medications intravenously. As they begin to take effect she will often be given oxygen through a large black mask that is placed over her face. She will feel herself getting a bit dizzy and drowsy before she loses consciousness. Then she will be given a muscle paralyzer. Since this affects her ability to breathe on her own, she is intubated—a long thin tube is inserted into her mouth, beyond her vocal cords, and into the main passage leading to the lungs. She will get oxygen and more anesthetic through this tube.

During the operation, the patient is tipped to her right side; pads are inserted under her left side to keep her in this position, which allows better blood flow to the uterus. Next, nurses wash the abdomen. The patient who is awake may be a little disconcerted to be able to feel the drops from the cleaning solution or the movement of her abdomen as it is washed (a relatively small area is deadened; areas close by are still capable of sensation). The woman is covered with drapes, and a small screen blocks her view of her abdomen. The doctor will check to see whether the anesthetic has taken effect.

Next come the incisions. The obstetrician cuts through skin, fat, muscle, tissue, and the peritoneum (the membrane that lines the abdomen); these incisions are called the abdominal incisions. The incision in the uterus itself is called the uterine incision. Each of these incisions can be made vertically and horizontally. Today the most common pattern is transverse (horizontal) incisions in both the abdominal layers and the uterus.

The type of transverse incision made in the outer layers is called a modified Pfannenstiel incision. Healing is better in this type of incision because there is less tension on the scar. Also, the scar can be nearly invisible since the incision is made below the pubic-hair line. The advantage of the vertical incision is that it is easier to do and takes less time. If the operation must be done

FIGURE 1

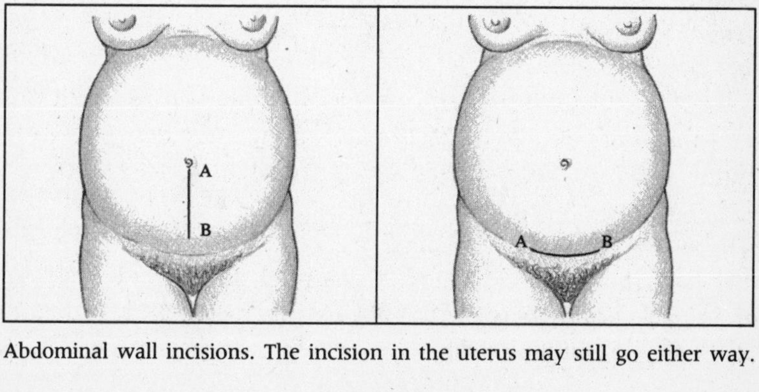

Abdominal wall incisions. The incision in the uterus may still go either way.

FIGURE 2

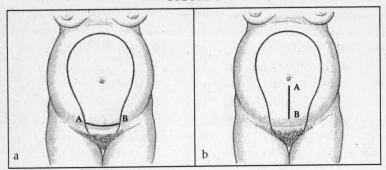

Uterine incisions: a) low transverse; b) classical

quickly (because the fetus or the mother or both are in danger) the vertical may be used.

Ninety percent of uterine incisions are what is called "low transverse." The uterus is cut in its lower segment, where the muscle is thin. The "classical" incision (a vertical incision) is made less than 10 percent of the time. It is more likely to rupture during the next pregnancy than a low transverse.

After the incisions have been made, the patient has lost about 150 centiliters of blood. The obstetrician comes to the amniotic membrane, cuts through it, and there's a big gush of fluid. The baby's head is usually the first thing visible. The doctor lifts the baby out. The placenta is removed by hand after the birth. There is quite a bit of blood loss during this part of the procedure. The patient is usually given a muscle contracting medication to try to reduce blood loss.

Then the obstetrician takes needles and begins to sew up the incisions: two sets of stitches for the uterus, one for the peritoneum, a few stitches in the muscle, a set in the fascia, a set in the fat layer, and clips or a set of stitches on the skin. The outer scar will be about eight inches long.

During this process the father can hold the baby so that the mother can see it. By then the baby usually has been cleaned and checked by a pediatric team.

Occasionally there are problems during the operation—most commonly difficulty with anesthesia, as in Mary Elizabeth Clinton's case, or exceptionally heavy blood loss. But in addition to the very small risk of serious problems, the patient will inevitably face certain complications:

She won't be able to eat for a day or more.

She will be in considerable pain and will continue to have some pain for about six weeks; she will often find it painful to urinate, defecate, or move freely.

She will have a catheter for a day or so.

She will probably need painkillers.

She will have a four- to seven-day hospital stay.

She will have a good chance of developing some sort of infection, which will need antibiotic treatment.

The cesarean is a relatively simple procedure, but it is major surgery nonetheless. In a scheduled cesarean with no complications, the woman doesn't have to go through labor, so in this way it is "easier." But the recovery period is typically longer and more difficult than for a vaginal delivery. A woman who places a high value on the emotional experience of childbirth may feel that a cesarean deprives her of that. Less recognized, I think, is that a cesarean can also deprive women of the full emotional experience of the first days or weeks of motherhood. A mother in pain will find it more difficult to enjoy and care for her new infant. Of course, the emotional experience can't be the final determinant. The doctor and patient must make the best decision for the physical health of mother and baby. Nevertheless, I believe doctors need to be (and many are becoming) more sensitive to the emotional health of the patient.

3

WHY CESAREANS ARE DONE

THE REASONS—
GOOD AND BAD

There are several major reasons why doctors perform cesareans. Although each of these diagnoses *can* be a legitimate reason for performing a cesarean, none should automatically lead to it. In describing the conditions that lead to cesareans, I will try to distinguish the vague symptoms that often result in cesareans from the serious problems that make the operation essential. I also want to explore the gray area, the area containing the cases that are not totally normal but that may nevertheless not need a cesarean. These are the cases that are most difficult for the doctor and the patient. I hope that by better understanding the various problems that can occur before or during labor, the patient can be a more effective partner in the decision-making process.

Dystocia—The Difficult Labor

Forty percent of first cesareans are done because of a diagnosis of dystocia. Since most of the subsequent pregnancies in these women will also result in cesareans, dystocia is directly or indirectly responsible for about a third of all cesareans being performed.

What is dystocia? Basically dystocia means a poor fit between mother and baby, making delivery difficult or impossible. But it's not as simple as "the baby is too big" or "the pelvis is too small." If that were the case, we'd be able to predict it, and we can't. The fact is, a woman could deliver a seven-pound baby by cesarean due to a diagnosis of dystocia and then, in a subsequent pregnancy, deliver an eight-pound baby vaginally.

Fit has to do not just with the overall size of the baby, but with where the infant is big; it has to do not just with size but with position—a baby facing toward the front is generally more difficult to deliver than one facing toward the rear. Fit also has to do with the woman's pelvis size, but it's not subject to measuring in any accurate way. The pelvis is an irregular passageway of bone and muscle. The doctor usually can't tell by a vaginal examination that a pelvis is too small. The records of most women who are diagnosed as having dystocia will indicate that their pelvises were listed as "normal" in vaginal exams during early visits.

So if dystocia has to do with fit but doctors can't predict it or corroborate their diagnosis with measurements, how do they know when a patient has it? We don't, really, but many doctors say a woman has it when labor is taking a long time or not progressing in a normal pattern. Clearly a long labor doesn't always mean dystocia. Plenty of babies are born after long labors; in the past labors of two or three days still frequently resulted in normal births. Today we don't let labors go that long, and that's a good thing, but there's still a great deal of variation in what's called dystocia. One doctor may make the diagnosis after six or eight hours and go to a cesarean; another may wait eighteen hours before making the decision; another may wait twenty-four and do a vaginal delivery. The truth is, we don't really know how many of our diagnoses of dystocia are correct, because we don't wait around to find out—once the diagnosis is made, the cesarean is performed, and there's no way of knowing whether the baby would have fit given a further trial of labor.

Genuine or absolute dystocia means that vaginal birth is impossible. If it is attempted it may result in injury to mother or child or both. Such situations are extremely rare, as I said. But they happen and can't be ignored in any discussion of dystocia. The small possibility of such a condition may make doctor or patient choose a cesarean. No doctor wants to let injury to the mother or child occur; no woman wants to go through it. Since we can't predict absolute dystocia, though, and since it's so rare, we shouldn't make decisions based on the tiny risk of it occurring.

To understand why dystocia is such a vague diagnosis, I think it's helpful to look at the history of the condition. Dystocia is one of the oldest diagnoses for problems in delivery. When doctors began making this diagnosis, there were plenty of genuinely misshapen pelvises around. The major reason was disease. Polio, for example, could result in a disfigurement in which the pelvic bones were so bent out of shape that delivery could be impossible. Very few modern women are subjected to the types of diseases or other conditions that result in severe distortion of the pelvic passageway. But eighty or ninety years ago dystocia was an accurate diagnosis. It was to women with this type of condition that Dr. Edwin Craigin referred when he coined the famous maxim, "Once a cesarean, always a cesarean." This phrase has been picked up and used for modern conditions, but it's irrelevant to most modern women. The very abnormal pelvis to which Craigin referred is quite rare today.

However, the diagnosis has survived. It has become a much broader one, a catchall, really, for any difficult labor that can't be accounted for with other diagnoses. For most doctors, dystocia now means, "This baby should have been born by now and I don't know why it hasn't."

There have been efforts to make the diagnosis more rigorous, to say, in effect, How long is too long? The two ways we try to get at this question are to consider length of labor and extent of dilation of the cervix. (During labor the cervix gradually shortens and dilates; it is fully dilated at ten centimeters.) Emanuel Freedman, an obstetrician, determined the time range in which 90 percent of all labors fall in order to learn what length of time could be considered "normal" for labor. There are time ranges for the latent phase of labor and for the active phase. (Latent labor begins with the onset of contractions that result in dilation of the cervix. Active labor usually begins when the cervix is about four or five centimeters dilated and dilation becomes more rapid—between one and two centimeters an hour. When the cervix is fully dilated to ten centimeters, the first stage of labor—consisting of the latent and active phases—is over. The second stage goes from full dilation to birth.) This distinction between phases is important. If a woman has had a very long latent phase, she should not necessarily be given a diagnosis of dystocia, since the capacity of the pelvis has not yet been tested—when the cervix is hardly dilated the baby's head has rarely descended far enough to let us know that the mother's pelvis is too small. It's possible that in the active phase, she may progress normally.

These numbers representing the length of time most women labor are simply guides, not absolute indicators of when labor can be termed abnormal. To be different is not to be abnormal. From twelve to twenty hours is still within the normal range for the latent phase. In some cases a dystocia diagnosis might be made before this point, but in most cases it should be made after the active phase of labor is well along.

The cervix dilates very slowly in the long latent phase of labor. In the active phase of labor there are also ranges of what the normal or usual rate of cervical dilation should be. If the dilation rate falls below the normal rate, it is called an "protraction" or "arrest" in the active phase. The patient is often given medication to try to get the process going again. These numbers for rates of cervical dilation provide another set of guidelines, an indication of what's normal; the doctor must decide if the case at hand falls far enough outside the limits to merit action such as a cesarean.

Time and cervical dilation are not unreasonable bases for a diagnosis of dystocia, but patients should be aware (and doctors should admit) that dystocia is now a diagnosis related to time and progress of labor, not to factors of "fit" that can be empirically demonstrated. A patient should know that the term cephalic-pelvic disproportion doesn't mean much. If she hears the term used regarding her labor, she should ask what is meant—that the cervix is not dilated enough? The baby is too large? (Is this borne out by ultrasound?) The patient should know what conditions the doctor considers to constitute dystocia.

RANGES OF LABOR TIME AND CERVICAL DILATION

Mean Latent Phase Labor Duration

0-2 cms.	9	27/60
2-3 cms.	7	46/60
3-5 cms.	5	22/60

In the active phase of labor, the average rate of dilation is 1.2 centimeters per hour for first-time mothers and 1.5 centimeters per hour for the others. Therefore the average time from 5 centimeters of dilation to full dilation is from a little more than three hours to about five hours. After full dilation, birth usually occurs within two hours for first-time mothers, one hour for other women.

Source: Peisner, D. and M.G. Rosen. "The Latent Phase of Labor in Normal Patients." *Obstetrics and Gynecology* 1985, vol. 66, no. 5, pp. 644–648.

Of course, every labor is unique and has to be judged individually. Having normal ranges as guidelines is helpful, but in real-life situations the doctor has to use medical judgment. If a woman is exhausted and incapable of helping with a vaginal delivery, the obstetrician may decide to go to a cesarean relatively early. That should be unusual. Treatments now include medication to relieve pain and to promote rest. On the other hand, if the case is falling outside the normal range, the doctor should be watching closely for problems, but I believe the woman should be given a chance to keep trying. Patients should be given support and encouraged to persist. Women should not feel that they must go to a cesarean in a long labor for the sake of the baby. Follow-up studies indicate that in births in which the diagnosis of dystocia was made, babies born vaginally fare no differently than those born by cesarean. There is no direct connection between long labor and problems in the baby. Certainly labors lasting days should rarely occur, but labors that last several hours longer than "normal" appear to be safe.

In cases in which there is a long labor and then other problems occur, it may look as though dystocia results in poor infant health. If there is fetal distress (indications the fetus is being cut off from the mother's oxygen supply) during a long labor and the baby is born with mental problems, was it a result of dystocia or a problem that had nothing to do with the length or difficulty of labor? It's possible an early cesarean would have changed the outcome; it's also possible the damage was there before labor. And damage can occur in a short labor as well as a long one. So I feel it's important to keep in mind that even if dystocia accompanied a bad outcome, it didn't necessarily cause it.

No one wants to frighten potential patients with accounts of outcomes that have very little chance of happening. Most—almost all—labors end in normal births. I mention the following possibility only because it is a factor in some doctors' decisions, but I stress that this is very rare. I'm talking about the situation in which the baby's head descends, or engages, and then delivery doesn't take place in the normal time period (two hours for a first delivery, one hour when the woman has delivered previously). When we say "engaged" we mean that the largest part of the baby's head has gotten beyond (below) the smallest part of the bones of the pelvis. To an obstetrician it means that there is room and vaginal delivery should be possible. Failure after engagement leaves unpleasant choices:

Forceps—in the old days we'd just put on the forceps and pull the baby out. This is a potentially traumatic procedure, and we like to avoid it if possible.

Vacuum extractor—a flexible cup is placed over the baby's head, a vacuum is created, and then the baby is extracted. This, too, is potentially traumatic.

The tincture of time—the doctor waits and hopes the baby will rotate or mold itself into a better position. The obstetrician can also use clinical intervention, such as manually rotating the baby, to try to improve the situation. A physician should be able to turn to such skills before resorting to a cesarean.

Even though failure after engagement is tense and difficult for mother and physician, it still usually results in a healthy baby. And the chance of it happening is so small that it shouldn't be a major factor in the decision of whether or not to perform a cesarean.

I can't fault any physician who uses the guidelines of normal time and dilation as determining factors in diagnosis and decision making. Long labors are hard on the mother, the doctor, and carry the small risk of being bad for the baby. Delivering vaginally may require good clinical skills and certainly requires patience and involves anxiety. It is also true that a great deal of difficulty in the active phase can foreshadow problems later on. I'm not advocating that we abandon the diagnosis altogether.

What I don't think is justified is the diagnosis of dystocia as a quick way to resolve a difficult labor. It's clear to me that this is what's happening. There is no other way to account for the increased percentage of dystocia diagnoses. It's true that babies are bigger, but so are mothers. The fact is, the diagnosis is made more easily and more frequently than it once was. If the increase in cesarean births due to the greater use of this diagnosis had resulted in a dramatic improvement in outcome, it would be justified, but it hasn't. The increased cesareans may avoid a small percentage of births that would have resulted in brain-damaged babies, but if labor is *causing* the damage, there will usually be some sign of fetal distress. On the other hand, the large increase in cesareans means many more women are put at a health risk and are put through an unnecessary procedure—without their physicians even knowing whether they are performing a procedure that will indeed prevent damage. Once again, prudent judgment is called for. The doctor must avoid extremes and yet act appropriately when action is needed. Understanding the very low incidence of the problem (not even one out of one thousand normal-sized babies is born with brain damage that could be related to labor) and the implications of the cesarean for the mother can help avoid the rush to operate.

Dystocia is a problematic diagnosis. There is no way to predict dystocia, and it can't be diagnosed until a good trial of labor has shown that there is some difficulty. Moreover, there is no clear-cut way to determine whether a particular difficult labor will endanger the infant or the mother. There are situations in which the diagnosis is justified and a cesarean is called for, but doctor and patient alike should know that in many cases it is not justified. If they can work together as an informed team, they can help lower the anxiety involved and reduce the chance of an unnecessary cesarean.

Fetal Distress

In 1986 one-third of the yearly increase in cesarean births in the United States related to the use of the diagnoses of fetal distress. This diagnosis is a major factor in the rising cesarean birth rate.

Fetal distress does not always mean exactly what it sounds like—that the baby is in trouble. In some cases it may be an indication that the infant is being deprived of oxygen and blood supplies and may die or suffer brain damage if not delivered quickly. But our ability to make firm, accurate diagnoses is limited. The words fetal distress only mean "a possible risk is present." Risk does not mean damage; it just means that the doctor must assess the situation and find a way to handle it. A fever in a sick patient is also distress. A rapid pulse is a warning sign in some illnesses. But these signs don't usually mean disaster. The term fetal distress is a frightening one. Some day we may have better terms and improved ways of learning when the baby is truly at risk and how damage occurs.

Several things can cause oxygen deprivation in an unborn baby. If the infant presses against the umbilical cord during delivery, or the cord is compressed in any way, or anything happens to cut off this supply line from mother to infant, oxygen loss can result. Sometimes the placenta detaches from the uterus (this is what happened to Mary Elizabeth Clinton in the case described earlier); here again the baby is cut off from the mother, this time at a different point in its supply line. When babies are not delivered by the forty-first or forty-second week of pregnancy, they sometimes outgrow the placenta. The placenta has a life cycle like anything else and begins to wear out, becoming less efficient in delivering nutrients to the infant. These post-term babies are at risk for fetal distress. If the contractions of the uterus are too strong or too long, that too can restrict the blood supply to the fetus and oxygen deprivation may occur.

If such deprivation occurs, it's imperative to get the baby delivered as quickly as possible. Unless labor is advanced to the point that a quick vaginal birth (perhaps a vacuum or forceps birth) is possible, that means a cesarean.

But as usual, things aren't as simple as they might appear. Everyone agrees that an oxygen-deprived fetus is in danger; but there is difference in opinion as to how we know when a fetus is indeed oxygen deprived. While we often worry about "possible" fetal distress, most times the baby is quite well.

The major tool for detecting fetal distress is the electronic fetal heart monitor. This machine is essentially a big mechanical stethoscope that listens to the baby's heart rate constantly and produces a two-dimensional picture of every fetal heartbeat and

FIGURE 3

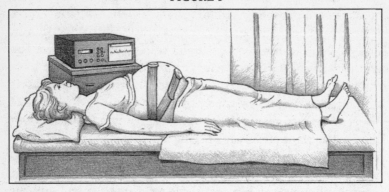

Electronic fetal heart monitor. Electrodes are in place on the mother's abdomen.

the resting periods in between. The doctor "reads" these tracings to determine whether the activity is normal or not. Most people have seen such tracings in a hospital or on television—a line interrupted by small peaks and valleys. The monitor picks up the heartbeat via electrodes, which are attached to the mother's abdomen. Certain changes in the heart rate are the clues to fetal distress, but every variation isn't an indication that the baby is in trouble. In fact, most changes are simply part of the normal variation that all humans experience. An increase in heart rate doesn't mean, in itself, that a fetus is having problems, any more than it does in an adult. My normal heart rate is 65; I can increase it to 130 or 140 by jogging. That increase isn't an indication of any problem, though—my heart is adjusting to my jogging by pumping blood faster because I need more oxygen and other blood supplies. The normal fetal heart rate is 120 to 160 beats per minute. Only by examining the nature of a change in fetal heart rate can we determine whether the infant is in danger. Sometimes the heart rate changes in conjunction with the contractions, slowing down with each contraction. These slowdowns, or decelerations, are quite common and usually are not an indication of a problem (although they can be if they are frequent and severe). A slowdown called delayed deceleration, on the other hand, is an ominous sign; it's an indication that the baby may quickly become oxygen starved. There are many types of variation, but only a few are strong signals of fetal distress.

Unfortunately, the diagnosis of fetal distress is often made following any unusual patterns in the tracings. Certainly since heart monitors were introduced the number of fetal distress diagnoses has increased dramatically. In some cases this has clearly saved lives and avoided brain damage. Yet the majority of the infants so diagnosed come out healthy, pink, and crying. Is it because the doctor caught the problem quickly? Or because there was never a problem? I believe in many cases the diagnosis is made when the condition is not present. Using the fetal heart monitor alone makes these diagnoses difficult and sometimes a judgment is a best guess.

There is a procedure that can be used to corroborate indications of fetal distress. It is called a fetal scalp blood examination. In this procedure a tube is inserted into the vagina. Through it the obstetrician can see the baby's head. The physician puts a tiny scalpel through the tube and nicks the baby's head, then inserts a capillary tube (a pencil-point-thin hollow glass tube) to collect a drop of blood. This is quickly analyzed for acid content. If the baby's blood is highly acidic, it's a sign of trouble. This acidosis, as it's called, occurs when the fetal system is functioning poorly because of lack of oxygen and the fetus produces acid as it switches to anerobic, or oxygen free, forms of metabolism. The fetus is trying to adjust to the problem. This same condition occurs in athletes who've exceeded their bodies' abilities to produce adequate oxygen supplies. Unfortunately, most hospitals don't use the scalp blood test—about 90 percent never use it or use it very infrequently. This is probably because it increases costs and is a procedure with which many doctors are not yet familiar. Most obstetricians rely on the monitor alone, but the two tests used together are better than either one used alone.

There's another clinical sign of a problem. It is the presence of meconium, which indicates there is fetal stool in the amniotic fluid. The fetus may release the bowel movement when stressed. But this isn't a reliable indicator, because meconium is not always present or detectable when there's a problem, and it may be present when there isn't a problem. It may be present in 5 to 10 percent of all pregnancies. It could indicate something that happened days or even months ago. In most cases it represents a transient event and does not show continuing fetal distress; babies born with some meconium rarely have problems such as brain damage.

I don't believe that the monitor can be a substitute for a doctor's medical judgment. Reading the tracings is still more an art than a science. There are certain patterns that very often accompany problems, but many times it's not clear-cut. How long does a pattern have to go on before there is a real problem? How much below normal must the heart rate fall before we know it's a real sign of distress and not simply a normal variation? The monitor simply can't be used as a diagnostic machine—so much variation and bing, we go to an automatic cesarean. The electronic monitor is, rather, a diagnostic tool, a source of information. If the heart rate changes, the message should be, "Watch closely." A small variation can presage a larger problem, but most of the time it's simply a blip that means nothing and goes away. Doctors should restrain the impulse to do the "easy" thing in such cases. Genuine cases of fetal distress usually make themselves known. Performing a cesarean on every case that doesn't tick away at a textbook-perfect rate doesn't help babies and puts more mothers at risk.

Although the monitor is the chief tool for picking up fetal distress, it is not necessarily dangerous not to be monitored. Remember that the monitor is really a big stethoscope. A human with a regular stethoscope can monitor a patient, too. In healthy women who have no risk factors, constant electronic monitoring is not necessary. I don't require all of my patients to be electronically monitored. Instead I keep a regular pattern of human monitoring—that is, someone listens to the fetal heart rate with a stethoscope every half hour early in labor and every fifteen minutes during active labor. The low-risk (normal) patient will do as well as if on a monitor if this kind of nursing support to "listen to" the heartbeat through labor is present (today we don't actually listen to the fetal heart; we use a hand-held ultrasound device that records the heart's movement during its beat and is made to sound like a heartbeat). As a matter of fact, many studies have shown that good listening, in an orderly way, is not only as good as the monitor in detecting fetal distress, but may avoid the excessive diagnoses that are more likely when we have every heartbeat and every contraction to look at. Sometimes too much information can lead to cesareans performed for the wrong reasons.

In addition, the monitor is cumbersome and prevents the woman from moving around. Some women see it as an unnecessary medical intrusion. I think they're probably right, for the most part. Just because we have a tool doesn't mean we have to use it all the time. I would want to deliver the baby of a high-risk patient—a diabetic, for example, or a woman with high blood pressure—with the monitor in place, but in most cases it's not necessary.

FIGURE 4

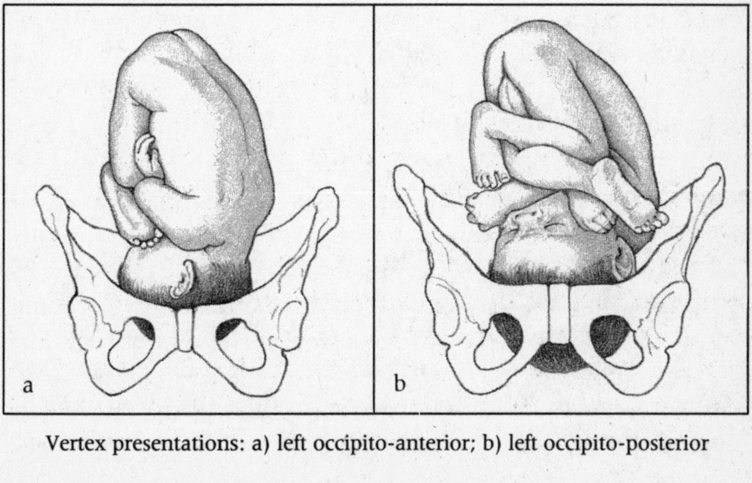

Vertex presentations: a) left occipito-anterior; b) left occipito-posterior

The Breech

The breech birth, in which the baby is coming down the wrong way, has always been frightening. The birth is often more difficult simply because the infant isn't in the optimal headfirst, or vertex, position. More worrisome, in the breech presentation the biggest body parts—the head and shoulders—come out last. In a delivery in which the infant is in the vertex position, the head is the first thing down, and since it is usually the largest part of the baby, the doctor can do a cesarean if it doesn't seem to be coming out. In the breech there's a possibility of having a half-delivered baby whose head or shoulders won't fit. That's a situation no obstetrician ever wants to experience.

It's not surprising, then, that the breech is one of the major reasons doctors perform cesareans. For many doctors, a breech position means an automatic cesarean. About 60 to 75 percent of breech babies are delivered by cesarean.

There are several types of breech. Two major categories are the frank breech and the footling breech. In the frank breech, the most common, the baby is in "cannonball" position: thighs flexed against the chest and lower legs bent against the thighs, with the backside down and presenting first. The footling breech means the baby is in a straight vertical position and comes out feet first. Although this sounds more straightforward than a doubled-over position, it is the trickiest, because it is the one in which the obstetrician can end up with the half-delivered baby whose shoulders or head haven't stretched the cervix open wide enough. Another type is the full breech, in which the baby is in a "jacknife" position.

There are certain problems that have been traditionally associated with the breech positions. One is the situation already mentioned, in which the head, coming last, does not fit. In this situation, injury to the infant and the mother can result. There is also an increased risk of the infant pressing against the umbilical cord during delivery. Breech deliveries require clinical skill.

FIGURE 5

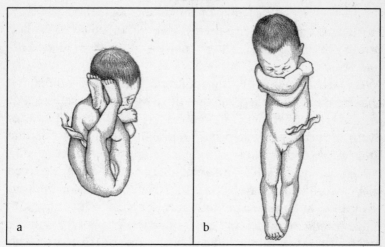

Breech presentations: a) frank breech; b) footling breech

For example, if the physician, during delivery, pulls the legs and body of a footling breech toward the ceiling with the head still in the vagina, the neck of the infant could be hyperextended and serious injury could result.

Because of these risks, the breech is likely to be delivered by cesarean, once again on the assumption that the cesarean is safer. Doctors feel that they have to get the baby out by cesarean because bad things tend to happen to breech babies. Bad things do seem to happen to breech babies: the mortality and morbidity rates are higher. But it appears that many of those bad things have happened before labor and, in fact, may be the reason for the breech presentation. Though at first glance the breech seems to be riskier—a straight comparison of vertex and breech babies indicates vertex babies have better outcomes—a more careful look shows that the breech is often not causing the problems. In studies we've done comparing brain damage rates of breech and vertex babies, we've found no significant difference in outcome if the comparison is done by weight. It turns out that many of the poor breech outcomes are not due to the breech position but to the prematurity of the baby; it happens that premature babies are much more likely to be breech babies. The problems of their prematurity far outweigh the problems of the breech—by tenfold, in fact.

Similarly, babies with congenital defects, particularly ones that change their physical makeup, such as hypercephalus (large head) or lack of kidneys, are more likely to be breech. Illness or death in such babies often has nothing to do with the fact that they were breech.

The footling breech is uncommon. The numbers are so small that we really don't have good statistical information on this type of birth, or on other, even more uncommon breech positions, to judge whether they are safe for vaginal delivery. For that reason, and because they can be difficult births, I wouldn't quarrel with any physician who routinely performs cesareans on patients whose babies are in the full or footling breech position. It may be that a sizable proportion of these could be delivered vaginally, but the supportive evidence just isn't there.

The frank breech, on the other hand, is more common and better understood. A great many babies that present in this position can be delivered vaginally. Unless it is a very large baby, I give patients with frank breech babies a chance to choose a trial of labor. Many of these women deliver vaginally; for those who have problems early in labor, we make the decision to do a cesarean more rapidly. The frank breech should not be an automatic cesarean. But this choice for vaginal delivery can only take place with the understanding and willingness of the patient. We have to explain all the problems just described here. We have to tell patients that most doctors deliver breech babies by cesarean, and this may make many patients feel that it's too risky to deliver vaginally. But it's important for patients to know that there is a choice in the case of a breech, and once more doctors begin to deliver some breeches vaginally, I think the tendency to automatically do a cesarean will be reduced.

Another aspect of breech birth that patients should be aware of is the fact that many, many babies are in breech position in the weeks before they are born. Most flip around to the vertex position before birth; a very small number flip after early labor has begun. There's no reason to decide on a cesarean before the due date if the baby isn't in vertex position, because there is a chance that by the time labor starts the baby will have shifted into the vertex. Further, about half the babies in breech position can be manually flipped around to the vertex. This involves a relatively benign procedure, called external version, done by the doctor near term but before labor. The obstetrician uses drugs to relax the mother's stomach wall and uterus. Ultrasonography helps the physician determine the baby's position. The abdomen is covered with talcum powder or oil. Then the obstetrician tries to coax the baby into doing a forward flip, pushing the mother's lower abdomen to get the breech out of the pelvis, then putting pressure under the head and rotating it forward, using the ultrasound picture to gauge the process of the manipulation. Sometimes we do this and the baby flips back to a breech the next day, so it's no cure-all. But about half the time we are successful. External version is a noninvasive procedure that can correct the problem of the breech. There is a slight risk that the umbilical cord will become twisted or constricted during the process, or that the placenta will separate; it should be performed in a hospital or environment with easy access to a hospital. This procedure wasn't taught in most medical schools five years ago; today more doctors are using it.

The Repeat Cesarean

Until relatively recently, the cesarean was a very risky procedure that was used only in emergencies. In the days before blood transfusions and antibiotics, the dangers of blood loss and infection were high. Since doctors didn't perform many cesareans, they didn't feel confident of their skills and so were less likely to use it as an alternative. From the turn of the century until the early 1950s, the rate remained about the same, around 4 percent.

As I mentioned before, the famous phrase "Once a cesarean, always a cesarean" was used by Dr. Edwin Craigin in reference to dystocia caused by diseases such as polio, rickets, and scurvy. Gradually, though, it came to mean that all women who'd had a cesarean must have subsequent children by the same method. When the cesarean rate was low, this practice didn't have much effect on the overall numbers, but as modern medicine made the operation easier to perform and less risky, the rate of first cesareans began to rise. Blood transfusions and the general availability of blood in hospitals lessened the dangers associated with blood loss; antibiotics made infection less of a problem; and training became more widespread. Once the base rate of cesareans began to climb, the repeat rate began to figure in. Today, with more than one in four births a cesarean, repeats clearly have contributed to the increase in cesareans, and they will continue to contribute at an ever-escalating rate. Currently they are responsible for about 30 percent of all cesareans. The myth is that all those repeat cesareans are necessary and that they represent greater safety for the mothers or their babies.

Because Craigin's phrase is glib and catchy, and because it fits with the idea that cesareans are safe and easy, it has become a maxim, accepted unthinkingly by many doctors and patients alike. I believe that the data do not support the idea that patients who have had cesareans should have subsequent babies by cesarean.

Over the past several years, I have compared postcesarean births to determine whether a vaginal delivery is indeed riskier than a cesarean for these patients. It is not.

The basic reasons given for the necessity of a repeat are (1) the danger of the scar rupturing, (2) the recurrence of the condition that caused the first cesarean, (3) the efficacy of avoiding an emergency cesarean; (4) the danger of infection.

Ruptures do indeed occur. But it's important to understand that the rupture is not like a balloon bursting. The scar rarely comes apart suddenly. The physician has advance warning—the woman has pain, there may be a bulge in the area, sometimes there are indications of fetal distress. I don't mean to minimize the rupture, but it is not something that's out of the doctor's control; it can be treated. Further, two-thirds of uterine ruptures take place *before* labor begins and thus before the date of a typical scheduled cesarean. The majority of ruptures doctors try to avoid by doing repeat cesareans will occur anyway before the operation can take place.

As for the argument that a repeat will avoid the conditions that caused the first cesarean—this is nonsense. In the large majority of cases, the difficulty of the first labor has no bearing whatsoever on subsequent ones. A breech in one labor does not mean subsequent babies will be in breech position, and, in fact, repeat breeches are uncommon. Among women who underwent a first cesarean following a difficult labor in which it was declared the baby couldn't fit, the majority will be able to deliver vaginally given a trial of labor, and of those half will give birth to a baby *larger* than the one delivered by a cesarean.

Some doctors say, "I can do a cesarean at thirty-nine weeks, the woman is in a healthier state, and it's much better than doing an emergency cesarean later." They may also point out that sometimes the woman doesn't go into labor at forty weeks and while the doctor waits, the baby could die. These are not good reasons. If they were legitimate reasons for repeat cesareans, they'd be legitimate reasons for doing a cesarean at thirty-nine weeks in all pregnant women. Not only would such a policy put mothers at increased risk, it would not even be safer for babies. Going to an extreme to avoid a small risk often brings on a new risk, and such is the case in trying to do cesareans before labor begins. We can't always predict due dates accurately, and if physicians start delivering babies at what they calculate to be the thirty-ninth week of pregnancy, we'll start to see more premature babies, no matter how careful we are. That is not a reasonable trade-off.

The possibility of infection is another risk factor in trying to let a woman who's had a cesarean deliver vaginally. If the woman gets into the middle of a trial of labor and can't deliver vaginally, for whatever reason, there is a higher incidence of infection than if the repeat cesarean were performed before labor began. An obstetrician can legitimately argue that performing a cesarean before the onset of labor avoids this risk. However, since *all* cesarean patients run a risk of postoperative infection, it seems to me more logical to attempt a vaginal, which carries the lowest risk of infection. Since most VBACs (vaginal births after cesarean) are successful, fewer woman will be exposed to the high rate of infection associated with both a scheduled and an emergency cesarean. In any case, such infections are treatable.

There are circumstances in which a scheduled repeat is necessary or advisable. Some hospitals lack the facilities to perform an emergency operation at any time of day. In many smaller hospitals, there is not an anesthesiologist available twenty-four hours a day; operating rooms and staff may not be available at all hours either. Here the physician's choices are shaped by the available resources. The obstetrician may have to perform scheduled cesareans because there is no guarantee that adequate staff and facilities will be available for an emergency operation in which minutes count.

Women who have certain types of illness may not be able to go through the stress of labor without endangering their health, and a scheduled cesarean is the best choice. (I will discuss such illnesses in the next section.) If a woman's previous cesarean involved a classical incision (fewer than 10 percent of cesareans), the risk of rupture is higher and the scar bleeds more heavily. We don't have good data, but I believe a scheduled cesarean is the wise choice in these cases. If the woman has already had two or more cesareans, we generally don't push vaginal birth. However, a few new studies have suggested that even in these cases choice may be appropriate.

These exceptions aside, most women who've had cesareans should be given a trial of labor. There aren't very many good reasons for the cesarean, and it causes additional risks:

- The pain, blood loss, and recovery put unnecessary stress on the patient.

- In some cases, multiple cesareans have long-term consequences, including abdominal pain, adhesions, and bowel obstruction.

- The necessity of blood transfusions increases a woman's risk of getting hepatitis, AIDS, or other infectious diseases.

- The woman misses the chance to participate in the vaginal birth, which for most people is a more emotionally satisfying experience.

- There are some complications that occur more frequently in women who've had multiple cesareans, including placental separation (usually fatal to the fetus) and placenta previa (the placenta attaches at the wrong place, making fetal distress during delivery likely).

- Women who've had cesareans tend to have smaller families (by choice) and thus it seems that some children who would have been conceived are not.

Finally, cesareans are more expensive. Some hospitals charge more, others charge the same rate for either birth route. But it costs more to do a cesarean and someone pays the bill. With rising medical and medical insurance costs, it does not make sense to be doing thousands of unnecessary operations every year.

These factors are not only reasons that the repeat cesarean should not be a norm, they are compelling evidence against the myth that cesareans are a safe, trouble-free way to have a baby. We can do them well, they are not extremely risky operations, but they are still major surgical procedures and can have major complications.

I know that for many women, the labor that preceded a first cesarean may have been a difficult and painful one. Some of these women tell me, "I had a horrible experience and was delighted to have a cesarean. I would never want to go through labor again." I would not try to force a woman who felt very strongly about this to try another labor, but I would try to make it clear that her experience the first time around does not determine what will happen in the future. Education for a vaginal birth after cesarean (VBAC) should start immediately after the cesarean birth. The patient should know all the things that happened during labor and delivery. The confusion and fear of the difficult events should be discussed; the physician should allay anxiety arising from uncertainty over what happened or could happen in the future. Finally, the patient should know that there is a very good chance that she can deliver vaginally in her next pregnancy and that she will be given an opportunity to try to deliver vaginally.

With the few exceptions I mentioned, I believe all cesarean patients who agree to it should be given a trial of labor. Women shouldn't be afraid of ruptures—they're rare and controllable. Patients certainly shouldn't believe that whatever was responsible for the first cesarean will automatically recur. Clearly "once dystocia, always dystocia" is not the case, since half the women who deliver subsequent children vaginally have larger babies. The same is true for breeches, fetal distress, and most other diagnoses that lead to a cesarean.

However, Craigin's dictum has become so prevalent that women who want to deliver vaginally may have to hunt around to find a doctor willing to let them try. I would like to see this change. When I attend conferences, I find that more doctors say they're open to vaginal birth after a cesarean, but I think the prevalent attitude on the part of doctors is still that the cesarean is safer and easier. This attitude is communicated to patients. Even if doctors say there's a choice, they often shade the discussion so that most patients will opt for a cesarean. The attitude should be that all previous cesarean patients are expected to deliver vaginally, that the vaginal delivery is the norm. This requires patients who are informed and willing to take a stand, and doctors who've been reeducated to put aside the old myth.

Other Factors

The four diagnoses I have discussed are the major ones for cesareans. They account for the vast majority of cesareans, and increases in each of these categories are responsible for the rise in cesarean rates.

There are other medical problems that can lead to a cesarean. I will discuss them briefly. A woman should be aware of these possibilities, but the likelihood of her encountering them (as opposed to the likelihood of her encountering a diagnosis of dystocia) is small. These categories include:

- postdate pregnancy;
- premature rupture of the membrane;
- placenta previa;
- various illnesses in the mother.

The Postdate Pregnancy

A postdate pregnancy means that the due date has come and gone and nothing has happened. It's important to remember that we still can't predict the due date with absolute accuracy. Why? Just as some babies grow bigger than others, some take longer to grow—they don't all grow at exactly the same rate. Some pregnancies end one or two weeks earlier and result in perfect babies; some take one or two weeks longer and also yield normal babies. So the physician may think the baby is late, when in fact the baby is right on its own schedule. Since no one knows what that baby's schedule is, however, we have to go on information that will give us a standard forty-week due date—the date of the mother's last menstrual period or an early ultrasound reading. If the baby is two weeks late by this schedule, we have to be ready to intervene, even if it doesn't turn out to be necessary. If we are fairly confident of the due date, we usually begin to watch the mother very closely if nothing has happened by the forty-first week. By the forty-second week everyone is nervous. The reason is that after term, the baby begins to outgrow the uterus. The placenta, the lifeline that brings in nutrients and oxygen and carries away waste, begins to age. It has a life cycle just like a human, and it gradually begins to function less efficiently. Eventually this can result in problems in the infant: There is weight loss and the skin wrinkles because the baby is losing fat. Our problem is that this condition is hard to detect, even with all our tests. We can try to get an idea from ultrasound, check for signs of fetal distress. But we have no reliable way of knowing whether this is happening or whether the baby is perfectly fine. For all we know, our forty-two weeks may in fact be thirty-eight weeks, for in truth the most common cause of a baby's going forty-two weeks is a false last menstrual period or a skipped period just before pregnancy. We (the patient and the doctor) made the error in estimating the menstrual period; the baby was right on schedule.

The choices are to induce labor, to wait for it to come by itself, or to perform a cesarean. I try to wait if there are no indications of problems. At forty-two weeks I will often try induction. If conditions for induction are not present, though—for example, if the cervix has not softened and started to dilate—our attempt at induction may not work. Stimulating the uterus with the chemical oxytocin, which is identical to the substance produced naturally during labor, can help tell us if the baby is in a healthy environment. If during the attempted induction the baby develops signs of fetal distress, we know the infant has outgrown its placental blood supply and needs to be delivered, and soon, by cesarean. If the baby shows no signs of a problem, we may let the baby stay inside the uterus, and a cesarean may not be needed. How long is hard to tell; both patient and doctor will often become very anxious, leading to a "let's get it over with" feeling that may make everyone more likely to choose a cesarean. This is the type of situation that demands all a physician's medical and emotional skills. A cesarean may be necessary, but patience and careful attention may make a normal delivery possible.

PERCENTAGE CONTRIBUTION OF EACH DIAGNOSIS TO THE OVERALL CESAREAN RATE

Previous Cesarean	36.0%
Dystocia	27.5%
Breech	8.7%
Fetal Distress	8.8%
Other maternal and fetal reasons	19.0%
Total	100.0%

[*Source:* Shiono, P.H., McNellis, D., and Rhoads, G.G. "Reasons for the Rising Cesarean Delivery Rates 1978–1984." *Obstetrics and Gynecology*, vol. 69, no. 5, (May 1987) p. 696.]

The patient who reaches the forty-second week of pregnancy is the exception; most women deliver long before. Few women will have to make the decisions associated with the postdate pregnancy.

Premature Rupture of the Membrane

If a woman's waters break (which means that the amniotic membrane, the sac in which the baby floats, has ruptured) before term, the obstetrician has a tricky situation. The doctor can simply wait and expect that a normal labor and delivery will take place, usually within forty-eight hours for the patient who is near her due date. The problem is that once the membrane is ruptured, the risk of infection is much higher and the chance of the umbilical cord slipping down, or prolapsing, through the cervix is greater. If the cord prolapses, the baby will press against it during delivery, shutting off the lifeline to the mother. The infection associated with the rupture is more problematic than postoperative infection following a cesarean, because in this case the baby is still involved, and its system can be harmed by the infection. Most women and babies do well if the doctor decides to wait; most often labor begins in one or two days. Unfortunately, because of worry of cord prolapse or infection, the mother usually needs to stay in the hospital so that a doctor can look for signs of problems. The inconvenience and anxiety can make waiting difficult.

Many doctors choose to induce labor, no matter what the condition of the cervix, very soon after the rupture. The argument for waiting is that once induction is started in these circumstances, the doctor usually has to try to finish it. That's because once contractions begin with the waters broken, infection is more common.

So the doctor ends up with choices: wait, which is difficult emotionally; induce—and then the clock ticks; or perform a cesarean to avoid the tension of waiting or the tedium of a long induced labor.

There's no easy answer to this one. If the rupture is very early, so that it's almost certain the infant will be premature, I would try to wait but watch the mother very carefully. If the rupture were to occur close to term, I might go to induction after a couple of days, or I might wait. To do this, though, I need the patient's understanding and help. It's too easy to just get things over with quickly by performing a cesarean.

Incidentally, for those women who are postdate or who break their waters early in one pregnancy, there is no reason to expect that it will happen again. The odds are that it won't happen in the next pregnancy.

Placenta Previa

I said earlier that there were very few "nevers" and "all the times" when it comes to cesareans. One of the exceptions is placenta previa. This is a condition in which the placenta is attached in the wrong place. Instead of being on the front, back, or sides of the uterus, it is attached over the opening of the uterus; that puts it right in front of the baby's head—and thus right in the infant's path as it moves downward in a vaginal birth. This positioning means that the baby will almost inevitably push against the placenta during birth, and bleeding, harmful to mother and baby, will take place. If the placenta is near the opening, the condition is called partial placenta previa. In this case, there may be room for the baby, so the doctor has the choice of giving the patient a trial of labor. In the case of a complete placenta previa, however, the diagnosis is straightforward and automatic: perform a cesarean.

FIGURE 6

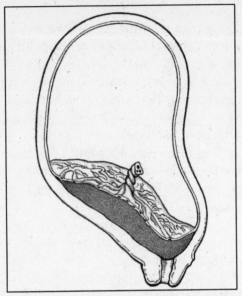

Placenta previa. The placenta blocks the opening to the womb. In this example, the cervix is totally covered and there is no choice but a cesarean.

Illnesses

Various illnesses in the mother can cause increased health risks to her or her infant during delivery. There is often room for judgment in these cases: If doctor and patient understand the condition and its possible consequences, there is often a possibility of having choices when the time to deliver comes. Following are some of the conditions included in this category.

High blood pressure. The risk is that it could get much higher during labor. In this case the blood pressure, if it is the only factor involved, can usually be treated. If the situation is complicated by other problems, such as possible kidney damage to the mother, the obstetrician may consider doing a cesarean.

Toxemia. This is a disorder we don't understand very well. It's usually of sudden onset, and symptoms include hypertension and albuminuria (presence of albumin in the urine), headaches, visual disturbances, and, in a few cases, convulsions. It can be life-endangering to the mother and puts the infant in a poor oxygen environment. Here, too, a cesarean may be necessary if the condition of the mother or the infant is growing worse, or if delivery will not take place quickly. Most patients with toxemia will tolerate labor and will deliver vaginally, but sometimes a cesarean will be necessary so that both patients can be treated quickly.

Diabetes. In some diabetic mothers, the higher blood-sugar levels are transmitted to the baby and result in increased insulin production on the infant's part. This in turn leads to rapid growth of the infant. It is just fetal growth in size, however, not maturity. Such a baby might reach eight pounds by the age of seven months, but would have no more maturity of lungs and other systems than the normal seven-month-old baby. These babies can grow quite large, and if they get too big, they have to be delivered by cesarean. However, this growth can usually be controlled by a careful diet and insulin regimen. If the diabetic woman consults an obstetrician before she becomes pregnant, or at least in very early pregnancy, she can be put on a program that will reduce the chances of rapid growth of her infant. Then she can deliver her baby vaginally.

Severe kidney disease. This makes the mother's system unstable and vulnerable to the stresses of labor. If the kidneys are failing and labor can't be induced, it may be necessary to deliver by cesarean. Once delivery takes place, the changes that pregnancy has brought to the mother begin to disappear and her kidneys don't have to work as hard; usually her system is then able to function better.

These are just some of the problems that might make the cesarean the better choice. In most cases in which the mother has health problems, she and her obstetrician will be aware of them and the possible consequences and will be able to discuss options ahead of time. For some of the other conditions, such as premature rupture, the woman won't be forewarned and a decision will have to be made fairly quickly. Women should be aware of these unpredictable conditions, therefore, so that if they should arise, they will be somewhat prepared and able to participate in decision making. I must stress again, however, that the chances of a pregnant woman having such a condition are very small.

Nonmedical Reasons for the Cesarean

This is a delicate area. There is a fairly widespread public perception that doctors do cesareans so that they can get to the golf course on time or so they have more money to spend when they get to the golf course.

It's undoubtedly true that not all cesareans are done from the purest medical motivations. But anyone trying to find out just how many cesareans are done for nonmedical reasons will find there's not much accurate data to back up allegations. Since most doctors probably don't acknowledge to themselves that they are letting time or convenience factors influence their medical decisions, they aren't likely to admit it to anyone else.

In what follows I will give my opinions as to how these factors fit in to the cesarean picture. I can't prove anything I say with statistics or studies; I can just say it comes from practicing obstetrics and watching others practice for three decades. It also comes from my general belief that people are basically good and try to do the right thing most of the time.

Doctors have been accused of doing unwarranted cesareans for several reasons: to make more money; to save time or inconvenience for themselves; to avoid lawsuits. I am going to discuss the legal question in depth elsewhere, so I'll just touch on it here. I will also include in this section some factors that I'll call pragmatic. They have to do with the resources the physician has available.

Money

Do doctors perform cesareans so that they can make more money? The federal government and Blue Cross and Blue Shield usually reimburse doctors and hospitals more for cesareans than for vaginal births. This is because the cesarean is more costly for the hospital—it involves a longer stay and requires more staff and resources than a vaginal birth. On the other hand, many doctors charge a flat rate for a delivery, whether it's cesarean or vaginal.

There is little data on this issue. There doesn't appear to be any significant difference between cesarean rates of doctors who can make more money from the operation and those who can't. Though some doctors do stand to make more money by doing cesareans, in my opinion most physicians don't do cesareans for that reason.

Hospitals and doctors who wish to eliminate the possibility that financial remuneration might be a reason for performing cesareans (or who wish to avoid giving patients the impression that the physician stands to gain by performing a cesarean) should simply charge a flat fee for all deliveries, vaginal or cesarean.

Convenience

While I don't think money is a factor, I do think that convenience sometimes plays a role. Imagine a delivery room where a woman has been in labor all night. The doctor sees slight irregularities in the tracings from the heart monitor. The physician also sees that it's 7:00 A.M. and thinks about the fact that patients are scheduled in the office beginning at 8:30 A.M. This makes it easier to weigh the scales of "possible fetal distress" or "possible dystocia" in favor of a cesarean; to make an early prediction instead of waiting to see whether problems are truly present. The obstetrician may very well write "fetal distress" on the chart and get ready for a cesarean. A doctor who's at the end of a long day, has pressing commitments, or is literally on the way to the golf course may choose a cesarean in a situation where labor has been fairly long or there are any concrete irregularities. Frankly, although I don't play golf, I too sometimes ask myself, Am I reaching a decision too soon because of nonmedical factors? There's always that underlying thought: I can get this baby out easily by cesarean and everything will be fine. And as the time of labor lengthens, I grow more anxious about the health of the fetus. This doesn't go away until I hear it crying. So it's a subconscious problem, but one that we should deal with correctly.

This convenience factor is particularly relevant to doctors in solo practice. If they are part of a group, they are on call in the hospital a certain number of hours. They can't go home any sooner if they do a cesarean, so there's not so much temptation. The data do indicate that resident services, where residents go home when their shifts are over, not when they finish particular procedures, run considerably lower cesarean rates than private services. I think that some of the difference has to do with the convenience factor, together with that comforting myth of the cesarean as an easy, harmless procedure.

In addition to the motivation of wanting to leave to go somewhere else, there's a more subtle way in which a doctor may be influenced to choose a cesarean for "convenience." It may not be that the physician has somewhere to go, but rather that the physician wants to get out of an uncomfortable situation. I'm speculating when I say that I think this happens frequently, but I do know that if the obstetrician is in the midst of an emotionally difficult delivery, there is a temptation to do a cesarean to end it. If the labor has been long and difficult; if the parents are emotionally distraught; if there are small but continuing fetal heart rate variations; if the patient is calling on you to do something or is asking for a cesarean—all of these make it hard to stick to your guns. The doctor knows the situation can be ended quickly, most likely with a good outcome. The doctor isn't trying to get out to go to a cocktail party, he is just wishing he could leave this situation and rest for a minute. I would guess that most obstetricians have felt like this, and probably many of them have chosen to do cesareans in some of these situations. It's not easy to do otherwise. Nobody can tell you how many points these factors contribute to the high cesarean birth rates because we don't know. I don't fault doctors for at times succumbing to the myth, but I do believe that patients and doctors can and should do away with the myth.

Pragmatics

The factors that I call "pragmatic" are ones that don't have to do with selfish concerns on the part of the doctor. Instead of making the best possible medical decision for the woman and baby, he or she is making the best possible medical decision given limited resources.

For the most part I'm talking about a doctor working in a hospital without the capability to handle an emergency cesarean at any time. A doctor in these circumstances may do a scheduled cesarean even though he or she would prefer to allow a trial of labor. If the hospital doesn't have a blood bank, an on-call anesthesiologist twenty-four hours a day, a pediatrician available round the clock, operating rooms or personnel available at any hour, then the obstetrician's choices are limited. If the labor progresses poorly and an immediate cesarean is necessary, the obstetrician simply may not be able to do it fast enough. This is a real concern. All hospitals should be equipped to give good pregnancy service, but unfortunately not all hosptials are. I'll discuss choosing a hospital in the next chapter, but the patient should be aware of the resources available to her doctor.

Malpractice

The last nonmedical factor that many people suspect figures into a doctor's decision to do a cesarean is the fear of being sued.

There's no question in my mind that this is a factor, and a major one. Most doctors will admit that this concern is always in the back of their minds as they make a decision as to whether a significant risk is present. Today, incredibly, most obstetricians either have been sued or know someone who has. Many obstetrician/gynecologists are dropping obstetrics or giving up their practices altogether because of the high insurance rate and the fear of being sued. Some can't afford to give up practice because they have to pay for insurance after they've stopped, since lawsuits may be filed years after a delivery.

As I've pointed out, the cesarean myths have taken hold in both the medical and the patient communities. Everyone seems to think cesareans are safe and easy and guarantee good outcomes. A third very important area in which the cesarean myth has been accepted is the courts. A prosecuting attorney holds up tracings from a heart rate monitor and says, "But, Dr. Brown, didn't you see these heart rate decelerations? Shouldn't you have diagnosed fetal distress and done a cesarean as soon as you saw these? Wouldn't we have a healthy child if you had?" I'm not trying to point the finger solely at the lawyers (who are after all doing their job)—the medical community is the one that promulgated the myth that we have the knowledge, the skill, and the gadgets to give everyone a safe delivery and perfect health for mother and child. And, indeed, the attorney can always find a physician who will testify that he or she would have acted differently. So doctors must accept blame for the problems the myths have created. The final result, though, is a legal system that perpetuates and strengthens the myths and forces doctors to practice defensive medicine. In many cases, I believe, obstetricians are performing cesareans not for the "safety" of the baby alone, but for their own safety. The cesarean is done to protect the health of mother and infant, but also to protect the doctor from legal vulnerability. Until we find an appropriate way to maintain patient rights for good medical care but do away with the huge financial risks and gains that come out of the courtroom battles, this myth that the cesarean helps avoid risk will persist.

THE UNDERLYING FEAR: BRAIN DAMAGE

I've discussed the diagnoses that lead to a cesarean, but we really need to know what those diagnoses mean. What are obstetricians afraid will happen if they don't step in and perform cesareans? There is more than one fear. The doctor who performs a repeat cesarean may be afraid that the woman's scar will rupture. The physician who avoids the breech may fear the rare situation in which birth causes physical damage to mother or baby or both. But what we obstetricians are most afraid of is delivering a dead or brain-damaged baby. And, though it may sound curious, the brain-damaged baby is often the worse outcome. As terrible a tragedy as the death of a child just being born is, it is a tragedy that fades with time. The family may very well be able to try again, to have a healthy child that, while it may never replace the dead child, can nevertheless bring joy back into the parents' lives. With a brain-damaged child, the pain doesn't ever go away; if anything it grows worse, as the child ages and the problems become more and more glaring. The death of a tiny child who only knew life in his mother's womb is terribly sad; the life of a twelve-year-old who's still in diapers and can barely speak is both tragic and enormously difficult for all concerned. The parents of such a child face years, often a lifetime, of emotionally strenuous and financially difficult care.

We can group brain damage into three broad categories: epilepsy, mental retardation, and cerebral palsy. These groups leave out conditions such as dyslexia and learning disorders. The reason I won't discuss such conditions at length is that we simply don't understand these disorders very well. We can speculate, but we can't pin them to something specific—is dyslexia due to a problem in pregnancy (probably not), a genetic condition (possibly), or some other cause? Since we don't know what causes them, and can't detect their presence during pregnancy or even very early in the infant's life, the lesser disorders do not figure in doctors' decisions about cesareans. The big three—epilepsy, mental retardation, and cerebral palsy—do figure in those decisions, however.

We know more than we once did about the causes of brain damage, although there are still big gaps in our knowledge. What we do know is this: While pure epilepsy and pure mental retardation are not related to events in pregnancy or labor, cerebral palsy can be definitely linked to such events. When I say "pure" mental retardation or epilepsy, I am simply trying to categorize these conditions as illnesses in themselves, distinct from their appearance as symptoms in other illnesses, particularly cerebral palsy. A cerebral palsy baby may have convulsions but is not suffering from the illness of epilepsy; another cerebral palsy infant may be mentally retarded because of damage done to the brain, but that is not the same as a baby born with mental retardation alone. The babies who have the "pure" conditions will generally look and move normally—their convulsions or retardation will be the only things that distinguish them. To the best of our knowledge neither of these conditions can be avoided with a cesarean or by any treatment during labor.

Some cases of cerebral palsy have been clearly linked to events during pregnancy and labor. Such events are not the only things that can cause it, but we know that they can. Cerebral palsy is not a simple illness, but a cluster of problems. Its manifestations are varied. The majority of those who suffer from cerebral palsy are not mentally retarded, though some are. Most are motor retarded, that is, they cannot control their muscles in order to move normally. The effects of the disease can range from mild to extreme. Some, despite their physical handicaps, can hold jobs, marry, and have normal children of their own.

One of the reasons the manifestations are different is that the causes can be different. Cerebral palsy can be triggered by genetic factors; it is often linked to premature birth; it can occur because of an infection during pregnancy; and it can result from fetal asphyxia, either long before labor, during delivery, or even after birth. In the very low birth weight or premature baby we believe that when asphyxia occurs it causes damage to the walls of the blood vessels, which may be only one, two, or several cells thick. These delicate walls then become like tiny sieves, and the blood begins to leak out. When this leakage occurs in the brain, the tissue is injured, there is poor oxygen supply, the wastes are not carried away, and the metabolism of the cells turns acid. In these circumstances, the brain is damaged. This phenomenon most often occurs in premature neonates, usually under fifteen hundred grams, or about three pounds. In such cases the damage usually occurs not during labor, but before or after. This theory is still not proven, and some believe that the lowest birth weight babies, if delivered by cesarean, will avoid this brain hemorrhage. The data do *not* prove that point at this time.

Clearly an obstetrician can't change a baby's genes and chromosomes by doing a cesarean; nor can the physician use a cesarean to deal with prematurity. We estimate that less than half the cases of cerebral palsy that occur (and perhaps only about a quarter) are due to events in the perinatal period (and that doesn't mean labor alone, but also the periods before and after birth). Let's remember, too, that cerebral palsy is rare—only two or three babies in a thousand will suffer from it. So one, perhaps two, babies in a thousand develop cerebral palsy because of perinatal asphyxia. Perhaps one of those cases of cerebral palsy could conceivably be prevented by a cesarean delivery. Right now we're doing about 250 cesareans to try to catch those one or two cases, and we *still* often miss the cerebral palsy babies. All we know is that if there are signs of severe fetal distress, damage to the brain can occur, but fetal distress is rarely severe enough to cause such damage. The asphyxia could occur because of pressure on the umbilical cord during delivery, because the baby is postdate (past the due date) and its environment is oxygen poor (the placenta wears out and doesn't produce sufficient oxygen and nutrition for the baby), and occasionally because the baby's environment is poor even though the due date has not yet arrived (such a baby is called dysmature, or growth retarded; it is not growing at the rate it should because, for some reason, it is not getting enough oxygen and nutrients). If we can detect these conditions early enough, we may be able to prevent brain damage. For instance, I delivered a dysmature baby who weighed about two pounds at thirty-four weeks—about half the normal size. We felt that the mother would not have tolerated labor well and that the baby was in more danger in the deprived fetal environment than she would be outside. So we did a cesarean, and it appears the baby will be normal. But it could have gone the other way—the brain damage could already have occurred by the time the infant was mature enough to risk delivering. Cerebral palsy babies don't always come with calling cards like dysmaturity. For most children with the diagnosis of cerebral palsy, there are no known risk factors that could have caused the problem.

In the field of obstetrics, physicians have worked very hard over the last few decades to understand and try to prevent brain damage. All of us hope we won't deliver a child with cerebral palsy, period. We do all we can to avoid it, because it's a terrible experience even in cases in which we're sure we weren't in any way responsible. If there is any doubt over the matter, we will suffer from guilt and remorse. It is one thing to witness suffering for which you are not responsible; it is quite another to watch sorrow that you may have caused.

But the fear of going through such an experience should not make us abandon strictly medical reasons for our actions. We're supposed to be professionals. Just as it would be wrong for me to assign a less qualified doctor than myself to do a surgical procedure on a patient because I was afraid of facing the family should problems arise, it's wrong for doctors to perform unnecessary cesareans. We do not yet have sufficient understanding of this problem to predict those few cases in which a cesarean might make a difference. Until we do, the only way to catch all such cases would be to deliver every baby by cesarean. The myth is that the cesarean will always prevent brain damage, and that it can guarantee a perfect outcome in every case.

4

RISKS OF THE CESAREAN

THE MEDICAL RISKS

In assessing risk for the cesarean as compared to the vaginal delivery, it's important to remember that both risks are very small. Prospective mothers should bear in mind that they have more chance of dying or being severely injured in an automobile accident than from any form of delivery.

The overall maternal death rate (death of any woman during pregnancy or within forty-two days of termination of pregnancy, due to a cause related to or aggravated by the pregnancy or its management) is now about 9 per 100,000 live births. When we consider that just fifty years ago the number was 582.1 per 100,000 births, we can see there's been vast improvement. Clearly we're better at caring for mothers. However, when we break down the statistic by birth route, we find that the maternal mortality rate for cesarean mothers is four times as high (40.9 per 100,000) as for mothers who deliver vaginally. Even for a scheduled cesarean, a woman is twice as likely to die as a woman going through vaginal birth. It's not that the cesarean is a highly risky operation—it's just that it *is* an operation and all surgery carries risk. Also, these figures show how very safe vaginal birth is. We've made tremendous improvements in handling the cesarean, but nature is still safer and more efficient than we are.

The numbers for the infant risk factors are more difficult to pin down. If we look at straight mortality rates for each delivery route, we can't find out whether the cesarean is "safer." It's presumably done, after all, in cases in which there is already some problem or risk. The question is, given the same set of conditions, can the cesarean be expected to produce a better result? Simply put, is it better for the healthy baby to be born by cesarean? Is it better for the at-risk baby? I've studied the data we have available, and I have not been able to discover significant evidence that cesareans produce better outcomes in most cases. In the cases in which I feel the cesarean is mandatory, the data show a significant difference in outcomes. So, for example, we know that if there is placenta previa (placenta attached over the opening of the uterus), the cesarean is substantially less risky for the baby; it will prevent problems that are very likely to occur if a vaginal birth is attempted. But in most cases—the gray-area ones we are most concerned about—the cesarean has not proved itself safer for the infant.

In addition to a mother's risk of dying, there is the risk of "morbidity"—any medical problem caused by the birth process or treatment during that process. The maternal morbidity rates for all birth routes vary substantially across the country, and because there are so many types of morbidity, we don't have exact numbers on overall maternal morbidity. Clearly, though, morbidity rates are far greater in mothers who have had cesareans. Complications typical of cesarean patients include operative injuries to the urinary tract and bowels, wound abscess, wound dehiscence (the suture line splits), operative and postoperative hemorrhage. As in any operation, there is a risk of anesthesia-related morbidity, as well as the danger of a blood clot in the veins, which, if it moves into the heart or lungs, can cause death or injury.

The most common problem is some type of infection following the cesarean; 20 to 40 percent of cesarean patients suffer infection. Infection accounts for 75 percent of the complications following the cesarean. In most cases the infection can be treated easily, but infections result in an extension in the average length of a cesarean patient's hospital stay. Women may have problems related to the cesarean weeks or even years later, problems such as unexplained pain or bowel obstructions from adhesions or scars caused by the infection.

No one should ignore these differences in risk. Those who tout the cesarean as a safe solution to everyone's problems ignore the fact that more mothers die when cesareans are performed and more women have medical problems following the cesarean than following a vaginal delivery. Maternal risks should be part of the decision on birth route, but they are not. Instead, we've tended to focus on the infant. The question has always been, "Is it better for the baby?"

If the answer to that question in a particular case is, "Yes, it definitely is better for the baby," than by all means we should perform a cesarean. But the answer is often, "Well, maybe it's better for the baby." We have still charged ahead with the cesarean. Finally, when the case is one in which a very minor complication has come up—say a tiny change in fetal heart rate, the answer is, "No, the evidence indicates that in cases like this the cesarean does not improve the outcome," but we've still tended to go ahead with the cesarean. It can't hurt, we've said, it'll mean we've done all we could for the patient.

I would advise those who would make the last two arguments to reconsider. If it's not going to improve the outcome for the infant, we certainly shouldn't be putting the mother at risk for no reason. And if it may help, but we're not positive, we must weigh that possible help to the infant against the possible harm to the mother.

I feel that it's vital to make these considerations. We can divide up the statistics for mother and child, but what we really should consider—what I tell my patients—is that the decision should be made in the context of a mother/child unit. They should be considered together. The question should be, What procedure gives us the best chance of producing a healthy unit, or an intact unit capable of recovering from problems that have occurred?

This conception is important. A woman who thinks only of her baby may not in fact really be thinking of the infant's long-term well-being. If a woman is told, "A cesarean poses some risk to you, but if we don't do it, there's a very small chance your baby will be damaged," and she responds, "Do a cesarean, I'll do anything for my baby's health," she's ignoring something very important. One of the most important things to any infant is the presence of a mother. If the mother does something that risks her own death or illness, she is also imperiling the health, physical and emotional, of her baby.

There's one final factor that is rarely discussed. Few consider what the cesarean means for the next pregnancy. I've been in the operating room many times confronted with a difficult surgery due to the scars or adhesions caused by a previous cesarean delivery. The placenta sticks to the wall of the uterus or bleeds more often in pregnancies following the cesarean, putting the younger sibling at greater risk.

While we don't expect the uterus to rupture, we are more cautious in handling women who've had cesareans. When labor begins, even prematurely, we worry more and deliver the next sibling earlier because we are afraid that the scar might rupture. Thus we end up handling the younger sibling's delivery in a less-than-optimal way because of the previous cesarean.

Like the other risks I've been discussing, this is a small one. A woman who makes a choice that's in the best interest of her whole family, however, will make the best choice.

THE EMOTIONAL RISKS—
THE EXPERIENCE OF
CESAREAN MOTHERS

When I began practicing, few people talked about a birth "experience." The idea of natural childbirth was not as widespread as it is today. Technology was considered to be only positive—no one talked about its down side. There was little concern over the use of drugs. If a woman was in pain, and sometimes even if she wasn't, the doctor was apt to give her some type of drug. Women learned about birth through other women or through experience, since few hospitals had prenatal classes. Women labored alone; the father was relegated to the waiting room for the birth of his child. When my first son was born thirty-one years ago, even I, an obstetrician, wasn't welcome in the delivery room (as it happens, I was in a different hospital delivering babies myself, so it didn't much matter, but the point is I would have had to look very hard to find a doctor who would let me be present at the birth of my child).

All that has changed—for the better, I believe. Families have come to value the birth of a child, fathers want to be there, mothers expect to be awake to experience the whole thing. Patients are prepared and educated ahead of time, since most hospitals now have some prenatal instruction. Because women know more about birth and value it, they also have high expectations.

The only drawback to all these preparations and expectations is that they are usually geared toward a positive experience, an emotional peak in the parents' lives. Not nearly so much attention is paid to preparation for disappointment. Rightly, prenatal classes don't want to scare patients with horror stories about what *could* happen. But the cesarean is no longer a rarity. In a typical birthing class, a quarter of the couples can expect to have cesareans. Most classes do have a session or sessions on cesarean birth, but the bulk of the preparation is devoted, as it should be, to the normal, vaginal birth.

Whatever the preparation, the inevitable corollary to the rising rate of expectation is a parallel increase in disappointment if events don't go as the family anticipated. Studies have shown certain feelings and emotions to be related to cesareans.

I want to describe briefly the emotional effect cesareans can have, as documented in studies and based upon my own experiences. I do not wish to make the cesarean out as some horrible, emotionally scarring event. Many women have no emotional side effects; some are frankly delighted with their cesareans. But the data and my experience indicate that the cesarean can be a source of emotional difficulty, and I believe the sense of failure or inadequacy that some women feel has increased as our society has begun to put more and more emphasis on the importance of birth.

Researchers have found a variety of maternal responses to the cesarean. These include fear of the surgery, of pain, of death, or of anesthesia; fears for the baby's well-being; feelings of powerlessness and loss of autonomy; lowered self-esteem; loss of feelings of femininity; change in body image with feelings of not being "whole"; jealousy of other women; difficulty in establishing feelings of closeness with the infant and in the "claiming" of the infant as her own; fears of another delivery; blame of the infant; grieving behaviors, including denial, anger, self-blame, and depression; and guilt at having these kinds of feelings at a time the mother believes she is supposed to feel happiness at the birth of her child.*

Most of the studies that have been done on the effects of the cesarean have been small ones. There really isn't comprehensive data on this topic. However, there are indications that cesareans do often precipitate negative emotional reactions. In a study of 105 cesarean mothers, 92 percent of the women reported feeling fear before undergoing a cesarean, while 50 percent reported dis-

*U.S. Department of Health and Human Services, *Cesarean Childbirth*, 1980, pp. 419–20.

satisfaction, anger, or depression. All the mothers vividly remembered uncomfortable preoperative procedures. All the women commented on the physical pain and difficulties of the postpartum period. More than half of the patients felt that their husbands had experienced disappointment, worry, and concern because of the choice of delivery. The majority of the women felt that a cesarean birth was harder than a vaginal.**

In another study in which cesarean mothers were directly compared to vaginal mothers (background variables, such as age, marital status, attendance of prenatal classes, birth weight and Apgar scores of the infant were similar), average labor was longer for the cesarean group, not surprisingly. Cesarean mothers in this experiment had less positive perceptions of the birth experience than did the mothers who had delivered vaginally. Women who had local anesthesia felt more positive about the cesarean than those who had general anesthesia. Cesarean mothers were significantly more hesitant to name their infants. They felt more hostility toward their infants, while vaginally delivered mothers were more likely to express concern for their infants. Cesarean mothers described the birth as a "shock," a "big disappointment," and "totally different from what I planned." Some felt that they had lost control, and these women were likely to express harsh criticism of themselves, their babies, and others. After birth, cesarean mothers were more likely to say they needed time to recover physically and emotionally before turning to the care of their new infants. They often saw the birth as "abnormal" and as a social stigma.†

Studies of women in the first months after birth suggest that cesarean mothers have more problems with physical discomfort and infant feedings and are more likely to feel anxiety and depression.

Whatever the short-term effects, there is not any strong evidence of long-term effects. One concern many woman have is

---

**Cesarean Childbirth*, pp. 422–23.
†*Cesarean Childbirth*, pp. 424–26.

the effect that a cesarean birth might have on bonding, the development of a tie between mother and infant that is believed to be stronger if the baby is kept physically close during the early hours and days of life. After the birth of her baby, the cesarean mother is still in the middle of major surgery. If there was a problem with the infant that precipitated the cesarean, the baby may be whisked away to be cared for. Even if the baby is fine, the mother may be groggy from anesthesia, in pain, or just restricted in movement (by IVs, drapes, and so forth). Of course, if she was given general anesthesia, she will miss the birth and the first bit of her infant's life. The average cesarean mother will be able to devote fewer hours to her infant in the first days following birth than a woman who has had a vaginal delivery. She will be experiencing pain, fatigue, and difficulty in moving around during the days following her operation. She is still a recovering patient, less capable of giving care. The concern about lack of contact is legitimate, although I don't believe that a mother who hasn't touched her infant in the first moments of life is forever handicapped or will never be able to form a meaningful relationship with her child. Also, hospitals are becoming more sensitive to the emotional side of delivery; more and more they allow and promote contact. Only in emergencies, when the mother or baby is in danger and must be cared for in isolation, is there any reason a cesarean mother can't have physical contact with her baby.

Studies also indicate that mothers fare better if they have a husband or support person with them during the cesarean, if they are awake for the operation, and if they are allowed contact with the infant quickly and are not separated from the infant for long periods. Again, most hospitals are becoming more progressive on matters like these, so some of the negative aspects of the cesarean are being alleviated by better care.

My experience pretty much parallels the findings of the studies. Patients of mine who had cesareans typically have a little more difficulty in adjusting than those who deliver vaginally. There's just no question that a successful vaginal birth is more fulfilling to most women than a successful cesarean. People seem to feel that there's an element of failure in a cesarean even if it was handled well and was clearly necessary. I have seen anger, guilt, and sadness over a cesarean. Quite a few women decide against having more children.

I don't want to emphasize these possible negative emotional consequences too much. Despite all the benefits of education on birth and the valuing of childbirth, such changes in attitude have sometimes created a climate in which the birth is overemphasized. It is important, certainly, but the child that results is the truly important part. I think it's unfortunate that a woman should feel like a failure for doing what was, or what she believed to be, medically necessary for the health of her child. Another reason that I don't want to overemphasize the emotional consequences is that they vary so much. Many women handle the operation with no problems whatsoever, many are downright pleased with it. The reactions that come in conjunction with the cesarean may have to do with the complication or crisis that led to the surgery rather than the surgery itself. Anxiety and disappointment may be due to a difficult labor as much as to the cesarean. I certainly don't want to suggest that cesareans should be avoided at all costs because they can be emotionally difficult. Patients should be aware of the possible negatives of the cesarean, but these should just be other factors to weigh. A mother cannot hold out for a positive birth experience when her baby's life is at stake. No one can indulge worries about possible damage to emotional well-being if an infant is about to die from lack of oxygen.

I discuss these matters mainly to help women keep perspective. A woman who is going through a difficult labor, or is tired and discouraged, or is being urged to give up her attempt at vaginal birth—that woman should remember that she'll probably have a more fulfilling birth and better aftermath if she continues with a vaginal delivery. She should remember that by ending her pain now, she only postpones it to the postoperative period; by giving in now, she may give up some early time with her new baby and bring on some emotional difficulties for herself.

5

PREPARATION

The final decision on what kind of delivery a patient will have is usually made late in the game. If labor progresses normally, of course, there is no decision to be made. If there are problems that the doctor thinks warrant a scheduled cesarean, the decision is made before labor. But many of the decisions to perform a cesarean are made in the hospital during labor. This is a highly emotional and stressful time for the parents. It's hard to make a calm decision when you're scared, or excited, or exhausted—yet this is often when the decision must be made.

The decision is often a difficult one, but it will be less difficult if the doctor and patient are comfortable with one another, have discussed possible problems ahead of time, and can work together. The woman who understands the terms associated with difficult births, who knows where her doctor stands on various issues, and who is able to trust her obstetrician's advice will be much better off when the question of a cesarean comes up in the midst of a difficult labor.

To that end, I am going to discuss measures a woman can take ahead of time to learn more about the process and to get the best possible match with her physician.

SELF-EDUCATION

We all have to be amazed that something smaller than the head of a pin (the fertilized egg) situated in an area not much bigger than the thumb (the uterus) ends up a seven-pound baby. It's a remarkable process.

It's also a remarkably safe process. The perinatal mortality rate (infant deaths that occur around the time of birth) in the United States is about seventeen per thousand births, eight to nine per thousand births for low-risk patients. The majority of these deaths relate to prematurity and to congenital abnormalities. These are very good odds, though of course to the families who experience the rare exceptions, the numbers mean nothing.

Pregnancy is not a dangerous condition. On the other hand, problems arise, babies are born retarded, babies die, mothers die. The important thing to know regarding the cesarean is that it can't fix most of these problems. There are things we simply can't avoid, no matter how good the care we give. For example, one of the major causes of death and damage to babies is prematurity. We have no way of controlling this. We are getting better and better at caring for tiny babies, but we haven't figured out a way to prevent premature birth. And a cesarean delivery will not add a day of maturity to an infant born before term.

Another area we do not yet have control over is genetics. If a baby suffers genetically transmitted abnormalities, we as doctors have no treatment to offer. A cesarean birth is clearly no antidote for a condition that was stamped on the fetus from the second it was formed.

So the first thing to recognize is that a cesarean will only make a difference in a small number of the small number of problem cases. Remember, though, that while only 17 of the 1,000 births result in infant deaths, about 270 of the 1,000 will be delivered by cesarean in the United States. Some of the 270 will have saved a baby's life or prevented damage, but we don't know how many. Some of the 270 will fail to prevent a problem in the child, because the problem was there before labor. Many will be unnecessary surgical procedures.

The patient should be familiar with the many diagnoses that can lead to a cesarean. When she hears her doctor say fetal distress, she should know what that term means. She should decide ahead of time whether she wants to keep trying under certain conditions, whether she wants to accept medication, when she thinks it's reasonable to have a cesarean. Such decisions may go out the window during labor, of course, since no one can predict what will happen or how doctor, patient, and infant will react. But if a woman has decided ahead of time that she wants to keep trying as long as there are no signs of fetal distress, it can make it easier to resist pressure—from a doctor, from family—to resort to a cesarean when there's still a chance of a vaginal delivery.

Another sort of mental preparation is necessary, too. Patients, particularly those who haven't been through labor, should understand that the process may be longer, more uncomfortable or downright painful, or more emotionally difficult than they expected. Nobody should come to the hospital terrified over the possibilities, but the patient will have a harder time handling a difficult labor if it's totally unexpected.

The patient should also know that she may need help in the form of medication. It's fine to go in expecting to avoid medication, but I feel there's no need to be heroic about this issue. If medication makes a vaginal birth possible and allows the woman to participate more fully in the birth of her child, it's worthwhile. The levels of medication given today do not have adverse effects on the infant, so accepting a painkiller is not going to harm the infant.

If the father is going to be involved in the birth, he, too, should educate himself. During labor, he has the advantage of a little distance. Since he's not in pain or carrying the baby, he can sometimes be a little more objective, though the truth is it's very difficult to be objective in dealing with someone who's close to you. Many fathers are more distraught during labor than the women going through it. But the father can give support to the mother, back up her decisions, sometimes help her stick to her guns. He may be able to play the role of intermediary between doctor and patient. He may be able to get more information on what's going on.

Just as the woman should consider choices she may have to make beforehand, the father and mother together should discuss various situations and how they want to handle them.

A few years ago I had a patient who showed up for her first visit with me with a five-page, single-spaced list of requirements. She had already been through a couple of obstetricians in this, her second pregnancy. She had had her first baby by cesarean, and it had been a bad experience. She was determined to have a vaginal delivery and she was going to control things this time around. She didn't want to be pushed around, and she wanted a doctor who would agree ahead of time to her list of very specific demands (she wasn't to be monitored under any circumstances, she was only to be delivered by her doctor, she wasn't to be given drugs, etc.).

She entered expecting an adversarial relationship. No one was going to make choices for her, but her way of trying to prevent that was to make decisions that can't be made ahead of time. No doctor should or can promise not to do a cesarean: In certain situations it's the only reasonable course. This patient had come to an obstetrician bound and determined to do everything possible to allow vaginal birth, yet she was demanding a promise I couldn't make.

I felt frustrated by her demands and by her confrontational manner. However, I also recognized that it came from bitterness over a bad experience. I knew she'd have a great deal of trouble finding a doctor who would work with her on her terms. I felt that her attitude opened her to the danger of having a second bad experience. I decided to try to work with her.

Her five-page list had to be negotiated like a contract: Yes, I can agree that you won't be electronically monitored, but if there's a problem you must submit to manual monitoring on a continuous basis; no, I can't agree to have your several family members and friends present because it's against hospital policy. We went down line by line. It was a tough process.

Six months later she delivered vaginally. I never completely won her trust; she viewed me as an adversary to the very end. Despite the vaginal delivery, she was still dissatisfied with the care she received.

That's how things go sometimes. But in most cases (including this one) they needn't go that way. Having been burned once, my patient was convinced a cooperative relationship involving trust was impossible. Had she been able to trust me, we could have worked together better and made the experience a very good one. As it was, she got what she wanted, but it wasn't a wonderful experience because she was tense and suspicious. The patient's goal should not be to control the process but to be involved in it.

There are doctors who make such a relationship impossible because *they* insist on maintaining total control over the process and refuse to let the patient become involved. There is one thing women can do about such doctors: find a new obstetrician. There is no reason any woman should be stuck with a doctor who refuses to let her have a role in the birth of her own baby.

The patient who finds a doctor with whom she is comfortable in the first place will avoid such situations. A strong physician-patient relationship in which there is trust and good communication is one of the best things an expectant mother can have going for her.

CHOOSING THE DOCTOR

The patient has the freedom to choose her doctor, and she has the freedom to drop that doctor if she's dissatisfied. I must qualify this a bit. Those who live in small, rural communities or are on certain types of health plans have more limited choices than city dwellers. But it's worth driving extra miles to a different doctor if a local one isn't satisfactory. Most health plans offer some choice, and patients should take advantage of that. I think it's worth a patient's while to make an extra effort to find a doctor with whom she is comfortable. The women who don't have the luxury of selecting such a doctor have to build the best relationship they can and be prepared to be assertive if necessary.

What's the best way to choose a doctor? It's not easy. The best way would be to see him or her in practice. That's usually not possible. A recommendation from a friend with similar attitudes about delivery would be very helpful, but that's not always possible either.

Most women have to get a feel for an obstetrician by talking to him or her. There are certain questions I'd suggest asking; their answers will provide clues as to the particular obstetrician's flexibility and attitudes. These questions regard a vaginal birth.

Do you electronically monitor all women, or can a normal, healthy woman do without?

Must I have an IV?

Will I be shaved?

Will I be given an enema?

Will I be permitted to move around during labor?

These are rather minor aspects of delivery, but I think they show a couple of things—first, how up-to-date the doctor is. Shaving the pubic area is out of the past, as far as I'm concerned. So is an obligatory enema (some people want one, and that's fine). Any doctor who forces these unnecessary procedures on patients is out of date (unless the hospital requires them, in which case you've learned something about the hospital rather than the doctor). The trend in obstetrics is to give a healthy mother more freedom of movement. Data indicate that it's better for the woman to be moving around during labor than to be flat on her back the whole time. Some doctors feel strongly about the need for a monitor, but the patient should look for some flexibility. Even if the obstetrician wants to monitor, can the patient periodically be unhooked and allowed to move around a bit? The answers the physician gives to these questions will give some idea of how flexible this person is in general. Is the doctor willing to accommodate you, or are there hard-and-fast rules?

Once you've gotten this far, ask the obstetrician what the limits of a normal labor length are. I consider eighteen to twenty-four hours normal, and as long as the patient wants to keep trying, I will let her continue for twenty-four hours or so before considering a cesarean. If the obstetrician says that labor shouldn't go on for more than twelve hours, then you know that this doctor may not want to give you time if your labor is long.

Next the patient should find out if the obstetrician has a set of medications used in all labors. There are several types of medication and anesthesia that can be used during labor, and some are better in certain situations than others. Further, the patient may have preferences; she may wish to have painkillers rather than an epidural. She may feel strongly that she doesn't want medication. Is the doctor willing to discuss alternatives, describe them, and allow the patient some choice in this matter?

Now you're ready to start finding out about the doctor's views on cesareans. If you have had a previous cesarean, want a VBAC (vaginal birth after cesarean), and hear those famous words ringing out—"Once a cesarean . . ."—you know you're in the wrong place. If the doctor says you had dystocia and therefore are too small for a baby to fit, you're in the wrong place. The previous cesarean patient should look for someone who's not merely willing to give her a trial of labor, but actively encourages it. You certainly don't want to hear, "Well, it's all right if you want this crazy thing." And "Well, it's all right" isn't that satisfactory either. You want to hear, "I expect you to deliver this baby vaginally."

For patients who have not had previous cesareans, the questions should be directed at finding out what the doctor considers to be the circumstances requiring a cesarean. Such patients also need to find out if the doctor has had experience in handling difficult vaginal deliveries. It's reasonable to ask whether the doctor has been trained to deliver a breech, or twins, vaginally. An obstetrician who has not is more likely to choose a cesarean. Ask the physician to explain a bit about fetal distress to you and to describe the monitoring process. You'll get some feel for how the doctor uses the monitor in this description of it.

Finally, you can ask what percentage of the physician's deliveries are cesareans. The response may very well be, "I don't have exact numbers," and many doctors don't keep track of this figure. But there will be a record of the hospital's rate, and if it is very high, it's a good bet the obstetrician's is high, too. While the cesarean rate alone does not tell you everything about the quality of care, it's certainly a start.

The answers to these questions should give you a good feel for the attitudes, flexibility, and temperament of the obstetrician. If you're satisfied with the answers, you've got yourself a doctor. If you feel the obstetrician is fencing with your questions, you should feel free to go elsewhere.

Once you have chosen an obstetrician, you should see this person as a partner. Ultimately, decisions about your health and the health of your baby will be in the hands of the doctor. Those decisions will be more likely to be ones you're comfortable with if you and your doctor have worked together from the start. This may sound trite, but I'm convinced it's a key to outcomes that are medically sound *and* leave everyone involved emotionally satisfied. It's in patients' best interest to be informed, but they should use their knowledge not as a weapon in an adversarial relationship but as a tool in a cooperative one. If the obstetrician thinks that the patient is simply waiting for a mistake to be made or views her doctor as someone out to mistreat her, that obstetrician is more likely to play it safe—and in today's obstetrical medicine, playing it safe means performing a cesarean at the slightest indication of nonnormal circumstances.

The patient should communicate to the doctor that she realizes there are no guarantees, even with the best of care, of perfect outcomes. She should indicate that she recognizes that there are unavoidable problems as well as avoidable ones. A doctor working with such a patient can relax, let the guard down a bit. The relationship can be a genuine partnership, with trust on both sides.

I don't know if it's possible to reduce either unnecessary cesareans or unwarranted malpractice suits by calling for a partnership between patient and doctor. I do know that in cases of my own in which I've had a good partnership with the patient, the results, good or bad, have been understood. Even when a patient who wanted a vaginal birth ended up with a cesarean, she didn't feel cheated, because she knew I was on her side, because she was part of the decision and felt it to be a necessary though regrettable one. In the case of a poor outcome, a patient who's worked with a doctor who took the time to discuss things with her is less likely to sue for a problem that was present before labor than a patient who was not part of such a relationship. I believe a stronger bond between patient and doctor can make a difference.

CHOOSING THE HOSPITAL

The choice of where to have a baby is a patient's right. In general, patients are good at finding places where they can obtain what they regard as good care; in general, hospitals that lose patients to institutions that better meet those patients' needs begin to change. But the patient needs to take some initiative so that she doesn't end up learning through an unhappy experience that a particular hospital can't meet her needs.

Here again I have to proceed with the caveat that some patients have more alternatives than others. Some women can't choose one hospital over another because there is only one hospital within reasonable distance, or because their health plan only covers certain hospitals or clinics, or because they have no insurance and little money and have to go to a hospital that will accept them. I can only repeat what I said regarding doctors: If you have a choice, take advantage of it; if you can get an alternative with a little extra effort, consider it. Those who have little choice still need to know what type of environment they will find themselves in when labor begins.

The major things to know about a hospital are how good its labor support is and what kind of maternal support environment it has.

The maternal support question has more to do with the emotional experience of birth than with the medical well-being of the mother. You need to know if the hospital has adequate resources to take care of you in an emergency, but I'll discuss that subject when I get into labor support. For now the question is, What will the environment in which the patient gives birth be like?

Many hospitals now offer the choice of a standard labor room or some sort of "home" or "birthing" environment. The labor room can be a single-, double-, or multiple-bed room, while the home environment is usually a single or double room. In both, the woman lies on a medical bed, but in the home environment, she'll be in a room that looks a little more like a bedroom than a hospital room. In some hospitals the entire family can come in the room, in other ones just the father. The woman can labor in whatever position she finds most comfortable. There may be several chairs, even a rocking chair, in the room. The major difference between the two environments is that in the standard labor room the patient is placed on a stretcher late in labor, moved into a delivery room, placed on a new table with stirrups, and will deliver in this operating-room-like environment. Today the delivery room is more likely to be used for more complicated births (such as a forceps delivery) and even for cesareans.

In the birthing room, in contrast, the patient labors and delivers in the same bed. If necessary, stirrups can be adapted to the foot of the bed just before birth. This type of environment is available for low-risk, healthy mothers in many hospitals. There has been a trend toward using birthing rooms more frequently— partly at the request of patients.

In addition to knowing about the types of rooms available, the patient should know whether there is adequate staff for her to have a nurse around all the time. Someone who's familiar with labor and can provide medical assistance is helpful, and the remarkable attachment that can grow between the laboring mother, her husband, and her nurse makes the birthing experience much richer for many. With the nationwide nursing staff shortage, many hospitals may not be able to offer one-to-one personal support throughout labor. And *any* hospital can have temporary shortages, since no one can predict how many patients will be in labor at any one time. Patients should find out what kind of nursing support is standard and how often shortages occur.

Some hospitals have rules regarding the use of monitoring, IVs, enemas, and so forth. The patient should know about these. She should know whether she'll be permitted to get up and walk around during labor, whether she'll be offered a choice in monitoring, whether she'll be required to have an intravenous infusion even if no problems are expected. Today routine enema use or shaving the patient should only be used at the patient's request or in the most unusual circumstances; hospitals where such practices are routine are behind the times.

The patient should know if the hospital has an education program for mothers-to-be (most do) and whether the program has sessions devoted entirely to the cesarean (many now do). Some hospitals have support groups for patients who've had previous cesareans—this is a good sign.

The area of maternal support is broad and loosely defined, but you should look for a hospital that is responsive to your needs and questions yet flexible concerning your desires. You should have choices in the matters I've been discussing, because these are largely issues of personal, not medical, concern.

The term labor support simply means the resources the hospital has available for handling various situations that can come up during labor. Ironically, the most important question for women who wish to avoid cesareans is, Can the hospital perform an emergency cesarean very quickly if necessary? If the hospital doesn't have such capability, a VBAC or a difficult vaginal birth becomes more risky. If the hospital can't get you on an operating table within minutes and be prepared to do a cesarean very quickly, it is more difficult for you and your obstetrician to make the choice of a VBAC—a scheduled cesarean would seem safer. Since in certain situations a few minutes can make the difference between life and death, health and brain damage in the infant, this question matters. The majority of hospitals that deliver five hundred or fewer babies a year will not have such capabilities. Any big-city teaching hospital will. The American College of Obstetricians and Gynecologists says that hospitals should have the ability to perform a cesarean within thirty minutes. Many but not all hospitals can perform an emergency cesarean and have the baby delivered in less than ten minutes.

The next question, of course, is, Will the hospital get you on the table too fast? What is the hospital's cesarean rate? If it is over 27 percent, it is over the national rate, which is itself unreasonably high. In hospitals with high rates, the tendency to go to the cesarean quickly is entrenched in the system. You will have trouble fighting it. Even if your doctor is sympathetic to your desires, it will probably be more difficult to resist the pressure to perform a cesarean than it would be in a hospital with a lower cesarean rate. I have recently heard from our former residents, trained and encouraged to perform fewer cesareans and allow longer labors, how difficult it was for them to be accepted by their fellow physicians, who felt their rates for cesareans were too low. There was no question of poor care, just a problem with low rates.

In brief, the patient should look for a hospital that has the technological ability to take care of her and her infant in any emergency but doesn't insist on using all that technology if there's no emergency. Also, the patient should feel that the hospital won't try to make decisions for her. This is always a delicate balance. The patient isn't the expert, after all. She may not be able to make the most objective or the best-informed decision and so should work with her doctor. But she has her role and her rights, and that's why she should try to choose a physician and a hospital that can meet her needs. She should only lose her role in the birth process in a severe medical emergency, and then only until the crisis abates.

6

THE DOCTOR'S DECISION

ETHICS

Making a decision during pregnancy or delivery is a unique medical situation. The physician is dealing with two patients in one body: two patients sharing a system, but capable of developing problems independent of one another; two patients whose interests usually, but not always, coincide; two patients with only one spokesperson.

Ethics in this two-patient system is a complicated matter. Usually, what's good for the mother is good for the baby. If she stops smoking, it benefits her health and that of her baby. If she is well nourished, her unborn infant will be well nourished. Although the fetus cannot speak for itself, in most cases the mother has her child's best interest at heart and thus is an acceptable spokesperson for the infant.

There are problematic situations, though, ones in which the interests of the two patients clash rather than coincide. For example, if the pregnant mother is very ill, the termination of the pregnancy by cesarean may be in her best interest (for example, a woman with renal disease whose kidneys are failing or who will be permanently damaged if the pregnancy continues). However, if the fetus is not yet mature, such termination may put it at risk. The doctor must decide whether to risk the woman's life by continuing the pregnancy or risk the infant's life by performing a cesarean before the fetus is mature. What if a cancer patient needs treatment that could be harmful to the baby? Again the obstetrician would be faced with a dilemma: Should the mother's life be risked by delaying the treatment to try to give the baby more time to develop? Should the fetus be exposed to such treatment? Or should the fetus be delivered and be put at risk for prematurity-related problems?

In trying to decide between the conflicting needs of the mother and child, the obstetrician may consider the quality and length of life of the patients. If the cancer patient is at great risk but also has a case that's so far advanced that she isn't expected to live for more than a few months, the doctor may decide whether to treat the patient at greatest risk or treat the patient who will, in a sense, reap more benefit from the treatment. The American College of Obstetrics and Gynecology suggests that doctors accede to the patients' and the families' needs and wishes in these cases. Not all doctors agree.

The cesarean figures heavily in the complicated ethics of pregnancy and childbirth because it often is an alternative the doctor must consider. If we were still back in the eighteenth century, we'd just have to muddle through a vaginal delivery the best we could, no matter what the situation. We've invented a lot of new technology and techniques, and the problem is figuring out how, and when, to use them. For example, what is an obstetrician to do if a patient demands a cesarean when a vaginal is possible and more desirable?

In an emergency, the difficult ethical decision will probably be made by the doctor. In other situations, the patient or family may be able to make the decision, or at least fully participate in the decision-making process. In an emergency or serious situation, I'll make a very strong case for what I feel is the best medical choice. If there is less urgency, I'll let the family decide, though I'll still make a case for what I think is the best choice.

In addressing difficult ethical decisions, I use my best judgment—and that always involves choices and uncertainty. The more knowledgeable my patient is, and the more she tells me, the better I'll be able to make the best possible choices when the difficult decision is mine. Patients should be aware of the kinds of choices that might arise so that they will be more able to make good choices.

DELIVERY ROOM DECISIONS

The birth of a baby is an emotional experience for all involved. For obstetricians and obstetrical nurses, seeing dozens or perhaps hundreds of deliveries a year, the mechanics become routine. But at least for most of us, the process still remains intensely emotional. The tension of labor and the joy of a birth remain real for me after three decades; the expression of love between husband and wife as they share their child immediately after birth still affects me. The tremendous strain of a difficult labor and the pain of a death haven't lessened over the years either. I've learned to handle such situations better over the years, I think, but frequently they still get to me.

I want to explain how emotional tension and the pressures of the medical environment can affect obstetricians and speculate on the effect that this has on the cesarean rate. We doctors may like to portray ourselves as cool professionals making decisions based on our study of the tracings coming from a machine hooked up to the patient, but the fact is, we may be greatly influenced by an overbearing relative, an exhausting night with an angry patient, or the terrible feeling of powerlessness one gets standing by the bedside of someone in great pain. We are trained to handle these pressures, but sometimes they affect us anyway.

I also want to show how obstetricians are influenced in their decision making by changes in medical practice over the last twenty to twenty-five years. I make different delivery-room decisions now than I did as a resident. Some of these decisions are based on improved techniques or new sensitivity; some are based on changed standards in medical practice.

Finally, I want to show the role of the silent threat present at every delivery: the lawsuit. Any physician who goes against the accepted practice risks making things harder in the event of a lawsuit. Notice I did not say that such a decision necessarily increases the chance of a lawsuit. I believe a doctor who presides over the birth of a brain-damaged child is likely to be sued whether that physician is incompetent or the most scrupulous and talented professional imaginable, whether that physician chose an early cesarean or went with a vaginal. Americans expect to have perfect babies, and they hold their doctors accountable if they don't. So doing a cesarean isn't really protection against being sued. However, it may provide some protection from a prosecutor's and a jury's perception of guilt. In our legal system, the doctor who did the early cesarean is presumed to have done all that could be done to protect the baby against damage. The doctor who didn't perform the cesarean, or didn't perform it early in labor, is more likely to be held accountable for any problems that developed.

We're humans, and we work in a flawed environment. We doctors bear part of the blame for the flaws, as I've pointed out, for doctors are the ones who convinced everybody that cesareans were so wonderful. But we are also caught in the system. How can I win in a situation in which the best medical decision I make may be labeled a bad decision in court and make it more likely that I'll lose a malpractice suit? Judgment means there were choices when the decision was made. There will always be doctors who will say in court that they—had they been there—would have acted differently.

For most doctors, though, there's a fear that looms larger than the fear of legal action. It's simply the fear of failure, of causing harm to another. We are trained to help people, and we expect to be able to. When we fail, or feel that we've failed, it's very difficult. We know that our decisions can have profound effects on the lives of our patients. Even a decision that was the best possible one under the circumstances can have a bad outcome. A few years ago I had a patient who had a scarred eye and forceps marks over the back of her neck. I knew that the very prominent and capable obstetrician who delivered her years ago would, if given a second chance, have delivered her by cesarean instead of going to a difficult forceps. But a doctor only gets one chance to act, and he does his best.

Today the cesarean myths have played to the natural concerns of the doctor and twisted them. They've made us believe we can escape unhappy consequences with a simple operative procedure, a procedure that's easier for us and, we've managed to convince ourselves, easier for the patient. A procedure that's safe, reduces risk, that protects the mother, the child, and the doctor. We believe all this, even though the data and our own experience tell us otherwise.

In the following cases, I've tried to show the difficulties of making decisions in the delivery room, of resisting the cesarean myths, of making the best possible decision when there's really no good alternative available.

Geraldine Donovan

Geraldine Donovan comes to me early in her first pregnancy. She's twenty-four years old and works for the phone company. Her husband, Charles, sells ads for radio. Mrs. Donovan is a comfortable patient, and her pregnancy proceeds without a hitch. Her eight-week checkup looks fine, and she tells me she's given up caffeine and alcohol. At twenty-four weeks, Geraldine and Charles go to a natural childbirth class. Charles often accompanies her to her checkups, and it's clear the two are a knowledgeable pair and that they should make a good working team for the labor.

About 10 P.M. on a Tuesday night during her fortieth week, Mrs. Donovan calls me to let me know that her contractions have started. Many first-time mothers are anxious to get into the hospital as soon as contractions start. They are often hurt or irritated when the doctor tells them to relax and wait a few hours. The first pregnancy—and for many people all pregnancies—may be a tension-ridden affair. I tell my patients they'll be more comfortable at home. They're more likely to get some rest and take some fluids at home. There's very little that can go wrong in the very early stages of labor, so the hospital and the doctor really aren't needed. Further, if it turns out to be a long labor, it will seem longer to everyone (nurses, doctor, patient) if the patient has been there from the first contraction. I don't have to say any of this to Mrs. Donovan. The minute I start to launch into my spiel, she says, "Relax, Doc. Do you think I want to pack myself over to Manhattan and spend the night with you when I could be at home with Charles?"

At about 5:30 Wednesday morning, Geraldine Donovan calls to say she thinks she's ready to go in. Her contractions are about four minutes apart. I tell her I'll meet her at the hospital.

In the screening room, we find that Geraldine is five centimeters dilated. She's come in at the ideal time; she's dilated the first five centimeters at home. Now the second five will be at the hospital—and these, the active phase of labor, are usually the shorter five. She has what we call a minus-one vertex. The vertex is the top of the infant's head, and we have standard positions that are given numbered identifications. Minus-one is still well up, but not abnormally so for this time of labor.

Geraldine labors steadily. She dilates right on schedule, about one and a half centimeters an hour. At the end of four hours, she's fully dilated, ready to start the second stage of labor. During this time she's been feeling fine. Charles Donovan is doing well as a coach, and his wife hasn't needed any medication. She's a low-risk patient, so I haven't been monitoring her electronically (I like to leave patients free to move around, if possible). In her first couple of hours, Geraldine padded around and wrangled with Charles over names, which they still haven't settled on.

About 9:45 P.M. she gets the urge to push. She begins to push and everything looks fine. We have what's called an S plus 2 vertex, not untypical for a patient early in this phase of labor. About five minutes later, a nurse comes and tells me that the fetal heartbeat was 80 to 100 after Mrs. Donovan's last contraction. This is below the normal fetal rate of 120 to 180. I think it's probably nothing to worry about, since occasional drops in the fetal heart rate are not uncommon and usually do not represent a problem, but I have the electronic monitor attached so that we can get a continuous reading. As we watch the tracings we can see that with each contraction the heartbeat is going down. The dips on the paper are not insignificant; this pattern is known as variable deceleration and is often associated with pressure on the umbilical cord or pressure on the head. We don't like to see much pressure in either place, but usually this type of deceleration is not a sign of problems.

Right now the baby's position is what we call left occiputo transverse—LOT. The occiput is the back of the skull. The infant still needs to rotate to the full anterior position—nose pointed toward the floor—that is the most easily delivered. Now the infant is looking sideways; it will take more work and pushing by the mother to make the baby descend further and face the correct way. The head has begun to shape itself to the pelvis as it should. Everything's fine—except this heartbeat is beginning to worry me. I have several choices.

I can do a cesarean. The decelerations aren't drastic, and I feel the baby is not in immediate danger, but there could be oxygen loss. If the baby comes out fine no one will even remember these decelerations, but if there's a problem, I'll see those tracings in court.

I can do nothing for the time being. My gut instinct is that this is not yet an emergency. I'd like to give Mrs. Donovan and her baby a chance for a normal delivery.

I can put on the forceps. This would be what's called a midforceps delivery, which nobody much likes to do. I think I can get the baby out, but using the forceps has become a stigmatized procedure.

I can do a scalp blood test. I am fortunate to work in a hospital that has the capability to do this test. It provides a second piece of evidence, so I won't be going just on the monitor readings.

I decide to do the scalp blood. I tell Mrs. Donovan we're going to insert a tube and use a tiny scalpel to get a drop of her baby's blood so that we can see if it's acidic—an indication that it's oxygen-deprived. "That's fine, Doc, as long as you don't make any tiny slips with your tiny scalpel," she says.

I do the scalp blood quickly. The decelerations are more constant and are getting me nervous. The results come back: The baby's blood is pH or acid level 7.3, absolutely normal. It doesn't seem as if the umbilical cord is being squeezed off, or at least not to the point of threatening the baby.

The decelerations continue. I think it's probably due to pressure on the head. I'm not overly concerned about that, since I don't believe such pressure can cause brain damage. I have to be somewhat concerned, however, since there is no certainty about this issue. I think I am right, but nobody gives me any guarantees in this case.

The situation is getting worse, too, because the baby's movement down toward birth seems to have stalled. Geraldine Donovan is pushing like crazy, with her husband supporting her back and the nurses counting out for her to try to sustain the push.

My guts are beginning to churn. I would like this baby's head to come down. It's now at S plus 3—still at what is considered a midforceps level. It looks to me like this is going to take another hour or so. The patient is working beautifully, but it's just going slowly.

The dips in the tracings continue. They look a little worse than before. I don't think I have an hour to spend; in fact, I don't want to take much longer. Despite the good scalp blood, I just don't like the looks of these decelerations.

I hate to turn to a cesarean, though. Mrs. Donovan is still going strong, physically and emotionally. I turn to the couple and say, "Look, the labor has not been going on for an excessively long time, but these slowdowns of your baby's heartbeat aren't good. I feel confident I can do the delivery with forceps. I'll have to give you anesthesia. Would you be willing to go along with that?"

The forceps have come to have a fearsome reputation. They aren't crude instruments that mash a baby's skull, but they're often perceived that way. It's certainly true that in the past we did much more traumatic forceps deliveries than we now would. With the increase in the cesarean rate, the forceps have become a rarity. Even though I think this instrument provides an alternative, I don't use it much. In this case, I think I should deliver the baby quickly, and I think I can do it without too many problems using the forceps.

Geraldine answers my question. "Do what you have to do to deliver the baby, Doc." We quickly prep while Mrs. Donovan is wheeled to a delivery room and given an epidural. As we head down the hallway to scrub, Charles Donovan asks me what the stuff on the monitor means—could the baby die? I tell him that as of now the baby is fine but that the decelerations could mean problems and that's why I'm working to get the baby out as fast as I can. "But could the baby die or be messed up?" he persists. "Yes, but we're not going to let that happen," I say, hoping I'm right.

In the operating room, a nurse hands me the forceps. The forceps is a two-bladed instrument. Someone described forceps as salad tongs the Green Giant might use. Geraldine has just been tested to make sure the anesthesia has taken. It has. She's tense, and so is Charles, who is gripping the edge of the table.

I slide the first blade into position. There's plenty of room between the baby's head and the pelvis. I slide in the second blade. Next, I lock them into position (this is more like locking a pair of pliers open than clamping down on something hard and locking onto it; it's done so that the forceps won't slip out of position).

I begin to pull. I find I need more pressure than I thought I would. If my heart were attached to an electronic monitor, the tracing would be heading up toward the ceiling. I know there will be forceps marks on the head. I think to myself, I just hope this baby comes out screaming.

Another pull, and the baby's head is born. I take off the forceps and reach into the baby's mouth to suction and clear her airway. As I do I feel the baby bite down, or gum down, on my finger. I relax. This baby must be fine. I put my hands on the infant and pull her free. Now we see the cause of the decelerations: The umbilical cord is wrapped around her neck, twice. But she seems fine and her Apgar is 8. It looks like the cord wasn't tight enough to do any harm, though we didn't know that before. In fact, umbilical cord problems like this are common. The forceps marks will be gone in twenty-four hours, and the parents are exhilarated. Geraldine is tremendously happy that she didn't have to have a cesarean. "I was sure that's what you were going to say when you talked to us before," she says. "I'm so glad we did it this way."

Charles Donovan shakes my hand and tells me that he's glad it's a girl or Geraldine might have considered naming her baby Mortimer. "I'm grateful to you, but not that grateful," he says.

Many doctors would have gone to a cesarean in this case. In slightly different circumstances—the baby a little higher, the mother more anxious—even I might have decided on a cesarean. Had I done a cesarean as soon as I determined the decelerations were occurring regularly, I would have saved myself a lot of aggravation. The baby could have been harmed had the forceps been applied poorly. I could have misjudged the difficulty of the forceps delivery (but had that happened I wouldn't have been forced to go through with the procedure, since I could have quickly switched to a cesarean at that point).

Despite all the ifs, I think I did the right thing. An early cesarean would have been easy for me but would have put Geraldine Donovan at risk, deprived the parents of a good experience, and produced a perfectly healthy baby who was in no need of such early intervention.

Chris O'Malley

Chris O'Malley has come to me in her third pregnancy. She has a history of very rapid labors. In the thirty-ninth week of her second pregnancy she called her obstetrician, a doctor at another hospital, and said she was having contractions and thought she was close to having her baby. Her doctor advised her to wait a few hours before coming to the hospital and try to get some sleep. He said there was no reason yet to call her husband, a construction worker. Two hours later Mrs. O'Malley was in the hospital, on the verge of delivering, after a frantic trip in a neighbor's car. She hadn't been able to get in touch with her husband in time and had ended up being taken by her next-door neighbor's sixteen-year-old son, who didn't yet have his driver's license and was as nervous as Mrs. O'Malley. The two of them had careened, terrified, the five miles to the hospital.

Mrs. O'Malley is understandably anxious not to let that happen again. I tell her that one labor, or even two, is not any kind of absolute predictor of the labors that follow, but that given her history I won't discourage her from coming into the hospital when she feels she's in labor, though I think she should try to stay at home a little while, since it's better to spend the latent phase of labor at home.

"Look, Dr. Rosen," she says, "I don't care what your medical books say, these babies come out of me fast, and I don't want to give birth on the expressway."

The pregnancy proceeds normally. Mrs. O'Malley's only real problem is her weight. She's gained thirty pounds since her last pregnancy, and gains rapidly during pregnancy, putting on almost forty pounds by the eighth month. It's not a serious problem, since she is otherwise in good health, but it does mean the baby is likely to be larger than her earlier babies.

In her thirty-ninth week Chris O'Malley calls me about 11:30 one Thursday evening. "I've started getting contractions."

"How far apart are they?"

"Oh, I'd say every six or seven minutes."

I tell her to come to the hospital and we'll check her.

In the screening room they find that she's just one centimeter dilated. Her contractions are not yet regular. The baby's head is quite high. At best she's in the very earliest stages of latent labor; the nurse who calls me to report says he doesn't think she's in labor, "but she's nervous as hell."

We wait a little longer to observe her. By that time it's 2 A.M. and I don't really want to send her home. Her husband, Dennis, drives home to get some things Chris forgot.

I check her again in the morning. No change at all. Still barely dilated, vertex still very high. Mrs. O'Malley says she didn't sleep that night. I ask her if she's feeling contractions, and she says no, not since late in the night. I tell her I think she should go home and get some sleep. I tell Dennis O'Malley to go to work but to call and check in periodically. Chris's sister, Susan, drives her home.

Friday night Mrs. O'Malley calls around midnight. She's confused. You'd think by the third pregnancy a woman would remember exactly what labor felt like, but no two pregnancies are exactly alike, and besides, emotions can confuse the situation. I can't really interpret what she says on the phone. I tell her to come back to the hospital. When she arrives, her condition is just the same, except that she looks very tired, as does her husband. I check her in and give her ten milligrams of morphine so she can sleep. She sleeps about four hours; Dennis O'Malley hardly sleeps at all. In the morning she's still at one centimeter with no change in the vertex. I could try to induce labor at this point, but there's no real reason. Her due date is still several days off. There's no reason to think she won't go into labor on her own. I send her home and tell her to sleep.

Saturday night my phone rings. Chris O'Malley is in tears. "I really think I'm in labor. I haven't been able to sleep with the kids here. Dennis is no help at all."

"Come into the hospital and we'll talk about it."

When she arrives her contractions are six to eight minutes apart. It's still hard to say whether she's in labor.

Four hours later, she's three centimeters dilated, and the cervix is about 70 percent effaced (shortened). The baby's head is still high, but that's common in the early labor of mothers who have had previous deliveries. It looks like she's finally in labor. Unfortunately, she's been awake just about all night, so I've got a patient who's already tired going into what I suspect will be a long labor. It's about 7 A.M. I decide to give her oxytocin, a labor-inducing substance that's given through an IV drip. I'm going to try to shorten the length of early labor.

By 11 A.M. she's at five centimeters. The oxytocin is working, but this still isn't going to be a quick delivery, I can see. Chris O'Malley is beginning to see that, too. Her concern had been focused on getting to the hospital on time for her delivery. Now she's beginning to be concerned about having a labor unlike her other two. "Why does this hurt so much more? Is something wrong?"

I tell her that everything is fine, it's just going slowly.

It takes her another two hours to get to six centimeters. (Normally a woman with previous deliveries dilates about one and a half centimeters an hour once she's reached five centimeters.) The labor is becoming emotionally as well as physically difficult. Mr. O'Malley made the mistake of pointing out to his wife that she'd often said she wished she could have had time to experience the births of their first two children and that now she was getting that chance. She's not speaking to him at the moment.

Chris reaches nine centimeters about 7 P.M. The baby's position, we can now see, is occiput posterior—the back of the head has not yet rotated to the anterior position, with nose pointed to the floor. That's no big problem, but it often means things will take longer.

At this point, I could easily throw in the towel. In fact, some doctors would have at five centimeters. I could say that this is going to be a big baby and she'll have trouble delivering. But I have no basis for saying that. The baby is large, probably about nine pounds, but not that large. At over ten pounds, I would begin to be concerned. The infant is still much too high for us to determine whether there will be a problem of fit. There are absolutely no signs of fetal distress—the tracings from the monitor could go into a textbook illustration of "normal."

I try to encourage my patient. I tell her she's doing very well. She tells me she's hurting like crazy and asks how soon it will be over. "There's no way of knowing, but you'll be fully dilated soon and then it usually doesn't take more than an hour." I give her some Demarol for the pain.

It's another two hours before she's fully dilated. She's irritated with me and with the nursing staff, but she and Dennis seem to be reconciled. They're both tired but seem ready to marshal their forces for the pushing. After an hour of pushing, though, there's no baby. In fact, she's not very close—the vertex is at S plus 2. But the head is low enough for me to see that it looks as if she can deliver the baby with no problem.

The trouble is, Mrs. O'Malley hasn't been pushing very well for the last half hour or so. She's just about crawling the walls in frustration. Dennis O'Malley is no help; he's stopped massaging her and coaching and is sitting in the corner. When I tell her it's going to take just a little more time, she says angrily, "You've been saying that for three days. Can't you do something? Can't you get this baby out, do a cesarean?"

She's put me in a tough position. Yes, of course I can do a cesarean, but I feel there's no medical justification whatsoever. The tracing continues to hum along, the baby's fine. She's been in the hospital a long time (more than twenty hours), but her labor is still well within the normal range. If I continue the labor now, we'll be exceeding the normal range of an hour for the second stage (patients with previous deliveries usually deliver within an hour of full dilation). But no one has proved to me that allowing this to go on more than an hour threatens the baby's health. I believe I should continue with the vaginal birth for a while longer. That's what I believe. What do I want? I'm tired, too. I've been up with this patient for three nights, and I've spent the better part of the day with her. She hasn't been the easiest patient to deal with, though the nurses are bearing the brunt of that, as usual. But she's beginning to get to me, too. Now she's given us an easy way out. Do a cesarean, she's saying. My nurses and I could be relieved of her in a short time.

It's not really an easy way out, though, particularly for Chris. She's not likely to tolerate the postoperative pain any better than she's tolerating labor. I don't think I'd really be doing her a favor, and of course I don't think it's right to do a cesarean when I don't have a good reason. On the other hand, I damn well better be right if I go against the patient's wishes. I look at the tracings—not the slightest abnormality.

"I want you to keep trying for another half hour, Mrs. O'Malley. I want you to try to help me as much as you can. Then, if you don't make good progress, we'll discuss a cesarean or other options."

"All right, but it's not going to do any good." She's now as convinced of this labor's interminableness as she was formerly convinced it would be over before she could get to the hospital. One of the nurses, Kathy Kann, talks quietly to Dennis O'Malley. He gets up and comes over to his wife. "Let's try, Chris," he says.

"I *have* been trying—" She pauses. "Okay. Half hour."

Now she's pushing well for the first time. The half hour is almost over, but she doesn't notice because she can feel she's making progress. The baby is born a few minutes later, at 10:50 P.M.

Chris O'Malley is now thoroughly exhausted. Her emotions are mixed. She holds her little girl against her chest and looks very content, but when I walk over to her she looks up and says, "I hope you're satisfied, Dr. Rosen."

Patients like Mrs. O'Malley make delivery room decisions doubly difficult. I've been doing this for a long time, but it's still hard to stand by and watch a patient who's in pain, who's frustrated, who's angry. If Chris had been more insistent in demanding a cesarean, I would have had a harder time. I still would have tried to persuade her to give it a little more time. I might have suggested she try to get the baby down the centimeter or two that would have put her in position for a low forceps. But if she hadn't progressed after the half hour, and if both O'Malleys had been insistent, I might have gone ahead with the cesarean. Certainly had there been any signs of problems, if the baby had been a little larger, or if there were irregularities in the heartbeat, I might have been more likely to grasp at such signs with Mrs. O'Malley than with a patient who was holding up well and wanted to keep trying.

What this kind of case shows is that the patient-doctor relationship is a symbiotic one. In theory we think of ourselves as the care givers, the professionals trained to give physical and emotional support to the patient. But the fact is we can't always do something to alleviate physical problems, and we sometimes find we can't give effective emotional support. The patient's response affects our ability to be supportive. We'd like for this not to be true. We strive to overcome our own emotions, but we're human. If a patient is hostile, unresponsive to me, or doesn't want to try to do what I'm suggesting, I'll continue to act like a professional and to be supportive in what I say and do. But let's face it, I won't be as enthusiastic about spending many hours in this patient's company. If there are indications for a cesarean, I may unconsciously seize them earlier or find them more compelling than I normally would. If, on the other hand, I have a patient who's in a long miserable labor but has continued to put her support and trust in me, I will find it easier to be supportive.

I suspect that Chris O'Malley will tell her friends that she was in labor for three days and her doctor stood by and did nothing for her. If she decides to have another child, she'll probably be as anxious and confused (or more so) as she was with this one. It's hard not to be affected by such patients. I wish I could have done something to change her outlook, that the birth had gone easier. But not every delivery is going to be a quick, happy event. Every woman should expect and hope for a great experience during the birth of a child, but every woman should also be prepared for a difficult experience.

Sally Schneider

Sally Schneider came to me for her first pregnancy. She was twenty-eight then, in good health, very bright. Her husband, Larry, wrote for a medical magazine. The two of them were exceptionally well-informed patients. Mrs. Schneider had a normal pregnancy. She called me frequently with questions and was occasionally anxious, but this isn't unusual for a woman going through the extraordinary experience of pregnancy for the first time.

Her early labor progressed very slowly, and things went downhill from there. She had been in the hospital for sixteen hours by the time she got to full dilation, and then nothing happened. The head wouldn't come down. Pushing wouldn't bring it down. Time wouldn't bring it down. Mrs. Schneider tried different positions; she labored on her right side, her left side, in the knee-chest position, even tried walking around. She kept trying very hard, though it was clear she was anxious and hurting. Eventually we began getting decelerations in the fetal heart rate. After a long, grueling process, we had to give up. We performed a cesarean and delivered an eight-pound, two-ounce girl.

I spoke with Mrs. Schneider the next day. She was exhausted, naturally. I congratulated her on her new girl, Rebecca, and we talked a bit. I like to mention the possibility of a vaginal birth following a cesarean as early and often as possible. The idea of "Once a cesarean, always a cesarean" has been so firmly implanted that I often have to spend a lot of time convincing women that a normal birth next time is possible, let alone that they should try it. So I said to my patient that despite the fact that she'd had a cesarean, there was no reason the next child couldn't be born vaginally.

She took one look at me, gave a brief laugh, and said, "There's no way I'm ready to think about having a baby again." This is a typical and expected response from a woman recovering from a difficult delivery. I told her that I just wanted her to be aware of the possibilities. She answered, "Dr. Rosen, I don't intend ever to go through that again. That was the worst experience of my life." I didn't press it. I just said I'd see her for her six-week checkup and asked her to please feel free to pick up the phone and call me if she had any questions at all.

I discussed the matter again with her on her six-week checkup. She let me talk but was resistant. Her attitude hadn't changed. It's easy to understand. She'd been through a very difficult process, one that left her traumatized. For most women the memory of pain, even in cases of difficult labor, fades over time. In a few, though, it just doesn't seem to go away. At six weeks it was also apparent that Sally Schneider was, in general, an anxious mother. For first-time parents, there's a large adjustment to be made. Everything changes: sleep habits, privacy, social habits. Their whole lives have to readapt to the needs of the newcomer. Some couples handle the transition practically effortlessly, others have more problems. Mrs. Schneider just wasn't comfortable around Rebecca; she didn't seem exactly sure how to treat her. She had a few specific questions on that visit. I did my best to try to give some general support and discuss topics that often are related to problems in adjusting. In the course of that visit we also discussed birth control during breast feeding, and Mrs. Schneider decided to use vaginal foam and condoms.

I didn't hear from her again until about four months later. She called, extremely upset, and asked for an immediate appointment. She said she thought she might be pregnant.

It turned out she was. She and her husband had been planning to have another child, but they'd planned to wait three years. The pregnancy was a shock. Although they never seriously considered abortion, they were ambivalent about the pregnancy. They were still having trouble adjusting to one baby; the thought of two was a bit overwhelming. For Sally Schneider, the prospect of another labor was terrifying. The experience remained fresh in her mind.

As the pregnancy progressed I kept giving her my spiel: The progress and outcome of one labor have nothing to do with the next; a vaginal would be better; if she had a trial of labor and there were difficulties, we could perform a cesarean. Her answer never changed. "I'm not going to go through that again. I want a cesarean."

If she had come to me as a first-time patient with this demand, I would have told her, "If you want to be sure of a cesarean, you should find another doctor, because I'll keep trying to change your mind." I feel strongly that almost all cesarean patients (with exceptions such as those with classical incisions, which are more prone to rupture) should try to deliver vaginally on subsequent pregnancies. Currently only about 10 percent of repeat patients do get this choice, yet studies show that 60 to 75 percent of repeat patients can have successful vaginal births.

Sally Schneider was already my patient, though, and had been for several years. I felt that I'd undertaken her care and should stay with her. I could have told her, "I don't do that," but she was having a hard enough time as it was. I felt I should stick with her to help her through a difficult time; I also felt, frankly, that I might yet convince her to change her mind. It's a delicate process, and I try my best to tread lightly. Talking about it upset her, but I felt I must bring it up. I would say to her, "I want you to consider trying for a vaginal delivery. I think you can do it. I'm going to continue to talk to you, but I want you to know the final choice will be yours."

The final weeks of her pregnancy approached. I put off scheduling the cesarean, telling her that we wanted to get as close to term as possible to avoid any chance of delivering a premature infant. What I was secretly hoping, of course, was that she'd go into labor on her own, come into the hospital and make good enough progress so that I could say, "You're doing great!" and then she'd decide to give it a try.

No such luck. The thirty-ninth week came and she pressed for a date. I gave her one. She came in, not in labor. I made my last effort at changing her mind. Her answer hadn't changed a word. "I'm not going to go through that again."

There was nothing more that I could say. This woman's emotional needs simply outweighed medical considerations in this case. I performed a cesarean.

I may have saved Mrs. Schneider, and myself, some grief. She could have had a second labor every bit as difficult as the first. I probably wouldn't have waited so long before operating, but it would have reinforced her unhappy feelings about childbirth. The cesarean didn't solve the Schneiders' problems. Sally is still an anxious mother; the two of them are still a little awkward in their transition to parenthood. But when I visited Mrs. Schneider the day after her son, Michael, was born, she was calmer and seemed more content than I'd seen her in many months. For her this was the right choice.

Patients like Sally Schneider are exceptions. Most of the blame for the high rate of repeat cesareans falls squarely on doctors' shoulders. In most cases we aren't even making women aware that they have the option of trying to deliver vaginally after a cesarean. Rarely are we doing what should be done—telling women we *expect* them to deliver vaginally and that the repeat cesarean should be the exception. Only occasionally is the repeat cesarean a problem created by the patient.

The typical situation, I think, is one in which the doctor makes it easy for the patient to choose a cesarean. For example, if I minimize the operation, downplay the longer postoperative recovery, and describe the cesarean as a way of "avoiding the possibility of your uterus rupturing," I would be playing on patient fears and not really leaving much choice. Although more and more women are now aware of the possibility of VBACs and are beginning to demand them, most patients still think repeat cesareans are perfectly natural, easier and safer than vaginal delivery. Their belief in the myth in turn makes it easier for the doctor to choose the cesarean.

The convenience factor plays a part here. A VBAC requires more out of everyone. The women has to come in as soon as labor begins and must be monitored constantly, so that if there are problems we can spot them early and handle them. The physician has to be there for the VBAC, too; he can't come breezing in late in labor and deliver the baby—he's there from the start. The cesarean, by contrast, seems easy. There are no obvious complications; it's quick; it can be planned; no one has to sweat over some tracings or worry about the rare rupture. It's no wonder doctors find it convenient to present the patient with little or no choice in the matter, and it's no wonder patients without good information, or ones like Mrs. Schneider who have good memories for pain, accept that.

If a patient senses that her doctor is not a strong advocate for vaginal delivery or realizes that she is being pushed toward a cesarean, she should consider looking for another doctor. Barring the exceptions I've discussed, there is no medical basis for discouraging the VBAC.

GOING TO COURT

Obstetrical malpractice suits are on the rise. In the last decade, there has been a large increase in the number of suits filed. Most obstetricians will be sued at some point in their careers.

In a survey conducted in 1987 by the American College of Obstetrics and Gynecology, 31 percent of all lawsuits against obstetrician-gynecologists related to the birth of brain-damaged infants. The average award for the obstetric claim was $221,000 ($643,000 in New York State). About 36 percent of all claims are dropped or settled without payment—these only involve anxiety and expense to the clinician. However, once a claim is filed, it takes about two years, on average, to complete the process. Nationally about 45 percent of obstetricians will refer high-risk cases (ones involving complicated medical problems) to superspecialists, in part to escape risky deliveries. More than 12 percent of the obstetricians in the survey had dropped obstetrical practice, at least in part because of their fear of lawsuits.

How does this fit into the cesarean picture? It changes patient care. And that is my gravest concern. Decisions are now being influenced by fear of lawsuits. Doctors are trying to protect themselves by choosing the cesarean birth route.

I've alluded several times to physicians' fears of how a certain action will be perceived and what questions will be asked should the delivery have a bad outcome that results in a court case. There is no hard evidence that the rise in cesareans is related to the rise in malpractice suits. It is just a general assumption and one that I share.

One study suggested that there was a connection, but studies of practice in settings where doctors are not open to personal liability suits, such as the military, have shown a rise in the cesarean rate approximately comparable to the national increase. So we can't say conclusively that physicians are doing more cesareans as a form of "defensive medicine"—doing them, that is, to protect themselves in the event of a suit rather than because they believe the cesarean to be medically necessary. However, we should note that a very large percentage of all malpractice cases involving childbirth fall into the categories "failure to perform a cesarean delivery" or "failure to perform a cesarean delivery early enough." A doctor who performs a cesarean avoids this category. My opinion is that while few doctors perform a cesarean solely on the basis of concern over possible litigation, such concern does help tip the scales.

I believe that the rise in the number of lawsuits filed is unjustified—but that's just my opinion. I have participated in a number of trials as an expert witness and have seen everything from very clear-cut instances of malpractice to cases that should never have been brought to court or even filed. Even had my experience been less diverse, it would be foolish to try to generalize from it. I'll leave that particular argument to someone else. I do think that some solution to the problem needs to be found, whether it be changes in the tort law, some sort of "no-fault" insurance that would guarantee all neurologically impaired children support and medical care irrespective of whether the problem could or could not have been prevented. If something is not done, possible legal suits will continue to influence the way doctors make decisions.

I would like to give some idea of what it's like to go through a trial as a physician defendant in an obstetrical malpractice case. Before I begin I want to emphasize that in focusing on the doctor's role I do not wish to minimize the anguish of a lawsuit for the parents who bring it, nor the anguish of having and raising a child with medical problems. No physician who has watched a patient cope with a massively brain damaged child, or has sat by an isolette containing a hand-sized baby struggling to breathe, can underestimate the emotional upheaval and pain that such parents feel.

I'd like to give the doctor's viewpoint not to try to put it on a basis comparable to the parents' but to show how the experience of being sued can affect practice.

The first fact of life for the obstetrician is that if there is a bad outcome, there's a very good chance that someone is going to be sued. Even if the problem occurred before labor, even if the physician practiced good medicine, there is still likely to be a suit. This is not because patients are money grubbing—far from it. The parents find themselves in a situation that is emotionally shocking and financially draining. They have questions; they feel guilt; they wonder how this terrible thing could have happened to them. And they wonder how they can possibly pay for it. Family and friends may tell them that they should sue. Under the current system, one can't blame the parents. The courts are the means available to them to try to solve their financial and in some cases emotional needs in such situations. The other factor involved is one I've mentioned before: the expectation of perfect results. Here, too, the patient can't be entirely blamed. We doctors have helped promote such attitudes.

At any rate, if there are signs of a bad outcome after a particular delivery, the obstetrician knows that there's a chance of going to court over this baby. Sometimes the damage is immediately evident: The baby comes out with a fractured skull following a forceps delivery. Sometimes the possibility of damage is there: The baby has a low Apgar score after a cesarean performed following signs of fetal distress. The baby may improve and have no lasting effects, or he may turn out to be brain damaged.

Often the problems aren't apparent right after birth. They may show up within six months, when the parents begin to notice that their baby is not developing at the rate the books say is normal or that their child doesn't look or act like other babies of the same age. The family pediatrician may notice these things, or have them pointed out by parents, and begin to test the baby, because this kind of delayed development often foreshadows cerebral palsy. Sometimes it's as long as two or three years before the problems become apparent or the bills begin to mount; a doctor can't really be sure for several years.

The obstetrician who has a poor outcome that's manifestly evident in the hospital may have trouble facing the mother. She is going through a period of terrible anguish, and about all the doctor can offer is a few words of comfort or a tranquilizer prescription, rather pathetic responses to such a situation. The doctor feels anguish, too, and may begin to second-guess the whole thing. Should I have induced at thirty-eight weeks? Should I have performed a cesarean? Should I have performed it earlier? It's already beginning to affect the obstetrician's medical care. The next similar case will be handled differently, whether for good reasons or not.

I should point out that in most cases the doctor is well covered financially. We have to be. When the malpractice rates go up, so do the obstetricians' fees, and patients as a whole pay the cost. The doctor's worries are emotional, not financial.

When the woman leaves the hospital, the obstetrician will follow the baby's progress if the child is in intensive care in the hospital, but the doctor is no longer medically involved in the case. Eventually the obstetrician has no more reminders of Mrs. Smith and her baby. They begin to fade from memory; the worry recedes a bit. It's possible for the doctor to forget, since the doctor is not the one facing the baby day in and day out.

After a few weeks, the obstetrician is probably thinking less and less about the Smith family. Then Mrs. Smith comes in for her six-week checkup. The obstetrician may feel hesitant about asking but finally will probably manage to awkwardly ask how the baby is doing.

Often the mother will say her baby is doing well. That's what she's being told right now. What this really means is "well for the circumstances." We still know so little about brain damage that we can't make any predictions. All of us have seen babies who looked like disasters at birth turn into perfectly normal children. All of us have seen what we thought were minor problems turn into major ones. Unless there is very extreme evidence of serious problems, nobody wants to make predictions about a baby, nobody wants to tell the parents that their child has a problem before they're sure.

The obstetrician, however, has gotten some seemingly positive feedback and is relieved. No more questions are asked, because deep down we don't want to face these things. Not all doctors are like this, of course. Some maintain close contact with their patients and face the problems head-on rather than hoping they'll disappear. But doctors are human, and we often don't do the bravest or best things when times are difficult.

Somewhere along the line that mother who said everything was fine realizes it's not. She sees specialists, has the baby tested, and continues to see signs that her child is not like other children. The bills mount. Relations among family members get more tense. It is not uncommon for couples to separate or divorce during these periods. The mother may begin to hear from friends and family: "You shouldn't be paying for this; it's the doctor's fault." Eventually the family contacts a lawyer.

The lawyer's first task is to see if the family has a reasonable case. The attorney will contact the hospital and begin to request records. The obstetrician who had let Mrs. Smith fade from memory is brought back to earth hard. Medical records, notes, and tracings from the monitor all flow out of the hospital and into the attorney's office to be studied. The hospital will notify the doctor that the records have been requested.

No matter how careful an obstetrician has been, there will always be holes. Perhaps the hospital has lost some information; the lawyer accuses the institution of trying to withhold data. During labor, the fetal heart rate was being checked every fifteen to thirty minutes, but there is a one-hour gap in the records. It's unlikely that of the 270-odd days of pregnancy that short time was the crucial one in which damage occurred, that there were no other indications before or after, but nevertheless it's possible, and the lawyer has caught an oversight. "But, Doctor," the attorney will say in the deposition, "isn't it a standard of care for the fetal heart rate to be checked every fifteen minutes in active labor?" Even if the heart rate was checked during that hour, if it wasn't recorded, it wasn't done.

If the attorneys decide there's a case, they will send a complaint, listing the "wrongful acts" committed. More records may be requested, and the medical staff members involved in the birth will begin to be deposed.

Deposition isn't a pleasant process. Some lawyers are very civil, but since it's their job to make the best possible case for their clients, they aren't there to be pleasant. They're trying to obtain information they can use in the courtroom against the doctor.

A nurse who was involved in the delivery may be deposed. She tells the lawyer it was her responsibility to take notes during the delivery. As the attorney probes, the nurse reveals, for example, that she had to pitch in when the doctor made the decision to do a cesarean because there wasn't enough staff present and there wasn't time to get another nurse. So, the attorney, says, these notes weren't written as the events described were going on? They were made a half hour after the baby was born? During the trial, the attorney may use this information to imply that the notes were written after the bad outcome was apparent and so may not reflect what really went on. But anyone who's seen preparation for an emergency cesarean knows that notes are rarely written then. Time is critical and the delivery takes priority until the risk to the mother and infant is over. This is not poor care; it's the real world.

The physician will eventually be deposed, too. The doctor will have to hire a lawyer, and that lawyer will try to prepare the doctor for the deposition, which often makes people feel as if they're under personal attack. Where were you born? What's your education? Have you ever failed a test? Have you ever been involved in a lawsuit before? Were you late to the hospital that night? Did you have an argument with your spouse before you came in? Did you have a drink at dinner that night?

The case is probably on the obstetrician's mind all the time now. It may make sleeping difficult. Everyone at the hospital knows; the nurses have all been deposed. The doctor may even wonder whether bad choices were in fact made during Mrs. Smith's labor. No matter what is done, the doctor is only right if the outcome is good. Everything else is second-guessed.

If the case goes to court, the doctor faces another ordeal. The parents will be there, clearly in anguish. They may testify; they may bring in their child. There will be another detailed examination of the physician's every action concerning Mrs. Smith. The attorney will ask detailed questions concerning those tracings, those notes taken by the nurse after the fact. Other doctors, expert witnesses, will come in and pronounce their opinions on the merit of the doctor's decisions. Today a medical expert can be found to testify for or against any medical action. I have seen leaders of our specialty assume opposite positions on a confusing case. I have also encountered many doctors whose opinions seem so bizarre that I can only believe they are influenced by the attorney who hires them.

Whether the doctor is found innocent or guilty, the process is painful. This kind of detailed public scrutiny is very difficult, even if the doctor is exonerated at the end. If there is a guilty verdict, it is shattering.

I know of one physician, a family practitioner, not an obstetrician, who had lived and practiced in a small town for thirty-five years. He had delivered two generations of many families. One of those families sued him when a child he delivered by forceps had brain damage. The jury concluded that he was not qualified to use forceps because he wasn't a trained obstetrician; but he had many years of experience and probably was as competent as any obstetrician. This man decided to pack it in. He said that he couldn't face a difficult delivery again, that he would feel too anxious about whether his actions were correct, that he would worry that regardless of whether they were correct, they would result in another lawsuit. He quit his practice and left town. It was his loss, because he could have practiced for several more years, and it was the town's loss, because losing a doctor is a loss a small town can ill afford.

It's easy to understand why any doctor who's been through such an ordeal may ask, Why should I ever risk putting on the forceps? Why should I ever hesitate to do a cesarean? Why shouldn't I do everything I can to prevent this from happening to me again?

We can't put aside the rising malpractice suit rate when we address the rising cesarean rate. Fear of being sued makes doctors practice more conservatively and try to defend themselves in advance. The courts have also shaped a new standard for what is appropriate care. This legal standard is different from the medical standard. We have a situation in which the legal standard is shaping the medical one, instead of vice versa. Partly because the courts say forceps are inappropriate and cesareans are appropriate, physicians avoid the former and embrace the latter. Difficult as it is, physicians must reassert their right to shape the medical standard and to shape it according to what our data and our experience tell us are the correct medical foundations for such standards.

7

CROSSROADS

There's no way to truly simulate a crisis. You can try to practice for an emergency situation, but a fire drill can never completely prepare you for a fire. The fire drill can help, though. You may discover a door that's supposed to be open is locked, that you took longer than you expected to get out, and so on. It may make you more psychologically prepared, since it's easier to handle a difficult situation if you've thought about it, prepared for it, and practiced for it.

To that end, I will present several cases. The reader will see the case from the patient's or from the doctor's perspective. In each case, there will be "crossroads"—points at which decisions must be made. The reader can make a choice, then discover which choice was made in the case and what the results were. No two cases are identical, but I think going through the decision-making process, realizing what knowledge is necessary, and what concerns must be weighed against one another can help.

PREMATURE RUPTURE OF
THE MEMBRANE

Sarah Riess is a twenty-five-year-old married woman in her first pregnancy. She is healthy, athletic, and outgoing. Her medical history shows no problems or abnormalities. She has been having a pleasant pregnancy; she had little morning sickness and felt wonderful throughout the early months. She swam almost every day and exuded the glow associated with pregnancy in myth more often than in reality. Even as she approached term she remained comfortable. She's a fairly large woman and seemed to carry the additional weight easily. Riess and her husband, Don Roth, have been taking natural childbirth classes and are looking forward to the birth of their child.

Sarah Riess's doctor is Jean Sims. Dr. Sims works in a group practice, and the couple understands that another doctor may deliver their child. Riess has met several of the other doctors in the group and is comfortable with the idea that Dr. Sims may not be there when she goes into labor. Roth and Riess live in a city, quite near the large teaching hospital where their baby will be born.

Early on a Monday afternoon, Riess, now in her thirty-eighth week, calls Dr. Sims. She's told that Sims is out of town for the day and will be back by early evening. Ms. Riess asks for another of the doctors. She gets Dr. Sam Zablonski on the phone a few moments later. She tells him she thinks her water has broken. Zablonski asks her to describe exactly what's happened. She says that a good deal of clear fluid has leaked out and run down her legs. "Sounds like premature rupture," says Dr. Zablonski. "Come on in to the hospital." A neighbor drives Sarah in; Don leaves work and meets her at the hospital.

Dr. Zablonski examines the patient. From what he can determine, it appears that the baby is near term size and in the vertex position. This is good news. It means the baby can be delivered right away, if necessary, to avoid the danger of infection that is associated with premature rupture of the membrane. The examination also reveals, however, that Riess's cervix is "long and closed." It has not started to efface (shorten), nor has it begun to dilate. Further, the baby's head is floating outside the pelvis. The infant is mature enough to be delivered, but labor has not started. It may start in an hour; it may not begin for another week and a half—there's no way of knowing, although it usually starts within forty-eight hours when the rupture takes place near term.

In addition to the danger of infection (which is a concern, but is also something that usually can be effectively managed), the premature rupture carries another risk: the prolapsed cord. This means that the umbilical cord slips out of the uterus or ahead of the fetus. If the baby's head is engaged, the risk of this is lessened, since the infant's head actually serves to block the gap left by the rupture and thus reduce the chance of prolapse. Since in Sarah's case the head of this infant is floating, the cord could slip down. The prolapse is a rare occurrence that is very dangerous. When labor starts and the infant begins to move downward, it will begin to put pressure on the cord. The result could be a dead or brain-damaged infant, although the risk of either is still low.

There are several alternatives Dr. Zablonski can consider: he can do an immediate cesarean; he can try to induce labor; he can wait and see if Sarah Riess goes into labor on her own.

Dr. Zablonski wouldn't mind doing a cesarean and getting it over with. He's just had a couple of patients with bad infections, and he'd feel a little more comfortable getting the baby out. Sarah and Don are very anxious to avoid the cesarean. They know from the prenatal classes and from discussions with Dr. Sims that there are other alternatives. Riess asks why they don't try an induction.

"You haven't even started the earliest phase of labor. You aren't dilated at all. I'm worried that if I try to induce it won't take or that you'll end up going through a very long labor."

Riess and Roth continue to resist the cesarean. They ask the service to see if Dr. Sims is back yet. The hospital calls her home, and her husband says she should be back in a few minutes. They wait, but she's still not in after an hour. Zablonski comes back and says that a decision must be made. Just then Dr. Sims calls in. She asks to speak to Dr. Zablonski. He comes to the phone and says, "We've got a premature rupture, term and vertex, but long and closed. I'd like to go in and do a section, but they're resisting."

"Look, I'd like to give her a little time," Sims says. "They really want the vaginal. Let's put her to bed, and if nothing's happened by morning, I'll try to induce. I can always go in for the cesarean if it's slow or if we get an infection."

Clearly, this is a gray-area case. There's no one right answer. Dr. Zablonski is right in wanting to try to avoid a prolapsed cord. Doing a cesarean won't altogether avoid the other risk, the risk of infection, since the cesarean itself carries a high risk of infection. He's just swapping one risk for another.

Dr. Sims is trying to be sensitive to the desires of her patient. She is taking a calculated risk, but it's a small one. She is making her decision on the basis of what happens most of the time, not on the basis of what can possibly happen.

Riess and Roth are right to speak up and say what they want and to get a second opinion. But they are patients, not experts, and first-time patients at that. They have much less idea of how difficult a long labor can be than does Zablonski, who's seen hundreds of them. Further, neither of them really understands what a prolapsed cord is. Don knows they discussed it in class, but he doesn't remember exactly what it is. Sarah remembers wrong. She thinks it means the cord is wrapped around the baby's neck. She remembers the leader of her prenatal class said that condition can be picked up on the monitor and almost always handled before it becomes a big problem. Neither of the parents asks about the condition; neither doctor fully explains it.

So, who's right? What should be done? Should Dr. Zablonski go on arguing, insist on the cesarean? Should he defer to the patients and their own doctor? Should they do an induction right away?

* * *

Zablonski pauses for a moment, then says, "Okay, Doctor." He hangs up.

He returns to Riess and Roth and tells them, a bit brusquely, that he's going to do one more exam before he leaves for the night, that Sarah is to stay in bed and avoid walking around, that their doctor will see them in the morning.

Riess is taken to a room. The importance of not moving around too much is explained. Nurse Randy Rodriquez helps her get settled and tells her to move as little as possible. "If you gotta pee, okay, but don't get up otherwise. Just buzz me if you need something. I hold the indoor hospital track record from the station to this end of the hallway."

Don leaves when visiting hours are over. "I'll be here in ten minutes if you need me—get Randy to call."

At 4:30 A.M. Rodriquez sees Sarah Riess's call button flash. He goes to her room and finds her standing at her bed, ashen, shaking. "There's something wrong. . . . I went to the bathroom and there's something, something purple. . . ."

Rodriquez is out of the room in a shot, calling "Lay down!" as he leaves. He grabs a nurse—"Stretcher to 201" and then gets to the station. "Notify a doc. Think we've got a prolapse in 201."

Moments later, Paul Dancer, a resident, is in Riess's room. Rodriquez and another nurse are there, shifting her from her bed to the stretcher. Dancer does a quick exam and then says, "Let's get out of here, OR 306." He puts his hand up Sarah's vagina and runs alongside the stretcher that way—he's trying to keep the baby's head from putting pressure on the umbilical cord, which was the purple thing Sarah saw when she got up a few minutes ago. Apparently she had gone into labor during the night, without being aware of it. The cord had prolapsed, slipping down into the pelvis. Now her baby was squeezing her own lifeline, pressing against the cord as she moved into the pelvis.

"Randy, call Don, call Don," Sarah is saying.

"Can't, baby. Got to get you to OR," he replies, jogging beside the bed and holding Sarah's hand as they careen down the hall.

Someone does call Don, and Jean Sims, too. They both arrive within fifteen minutes. It's all over by then. Dancer had the baby delivered ten minutes after he was called. He is already starting to sew Sarah's incision. The pediatricians are working furiously on the little girl. She was limp when she came out, with an Apgar score of three. Sims comes and talks to Roth briefly, then takes Riess's chart and reads it. Suddenly she exclaims, "God-damn it, nobody told me the head was floating! Why didn't Zablonski tell me that?"

It's a messy case. Sims is angry with Zablonski for not mention-ing the fact that the baby's head wasn't engaged, but the fact is, she should have asked. She may think in retrospect—after the emergency has happened—that she would have made a different decision, but she might not have. Dr. Zablonski is defensive about the case. He lets it be known that he had wanted to do a cesarean in the first place. But if he had been so convinced he was right he should have gone ahead and done it, rather than waiting, and he certainly should have argued more vigorously. He was remiss for not fully explaining the case to Sims. The fact is, if the child had been born healthy after a normal delivery, he would have forgotten the incident the next day.

Riess and Roth now blame the hospital and the two doctors for not making the risk clear and explaining exactly what a pro-lapsed cord meant. But they feel a bit of guilt, too. They argued forcefully against Dr. Zablonski. Don, in particular, agonizes over the fact that he never just asked what the term "prolapsed cord" meant.

Both doctors' responses were reasonable. The parents' desire for a vaginal birth was reasonable. Things would have been bet-ter had communication been better, but nothing medically im-proper was done.

A prolapsed cord happens rarely, but it is a risk involved with waiting for a vaginal delivery rather than doing a cesarean after a premature rupture. As I've tried to point out, though, there's a risk involved in every decision. When one risk is very great and one very small, the decision is easy. But when two very small risks are involved it's more difficult. It's a bit like weighing the risks associated with sugar against those associated with artificial sweeteners. Both may involve very small risk of reducing life expectancy—a few days perhaps in both cases. Most people wouldn't consider a few added days of life expectancy grounds for choosing one sweetener over the other. They would make the decision for other reasons. I argue that the same applies to many cases in obstetrics. Playing a numbers game seems logical. Just do what's less risky. But when both risks are tiny, the numbers become less meaningful.

Of course, they may not seem so in court. Let's say that within six months it's apparent that Sarah's baby, Sharon, has suffered some brain damage. If Riess and Roth go to court, the jury very well may decide that they weren't properly informed of risk, that the doctors acted negligently in not doing a cesarean.

If so, Dr. Sims will practice more like Dr. Zablonski in the future. Dr. Zablonski will become even more conservative. The cesarean rate of the hospital will probably go up. The spiral toward unreasonably high rates will continue.

LARGE BABIES

Dr. Michael Miner is an obstetrician at a county hospital in a large city. More than half the obstetrical patients he sees are teenagers, almost all unmarried.

Jesse White is one of them—she's nineteen, unmarried, with two children and a third on the way. Jesse's boyfriend is the father of all three; the two have been a couple since Jesse was twelve. Jesse lives with her mother, Mrs. Janice White, who supports all of them with her job as a secretary. The boyfriend,

John, is unemployed. He plays with the kids when he's around, Jesse says, but he's not around much. Once she brought him in for one of her appointments, at Miner's urging. John sat silent and uncomfortable the whole time.

Mrs. White, on the other hand, always has plenty to say. She calls Miner quite often to tell him what she thinks he should be doing for her daughter. She approves of some of his advice—he's convinced Jesse to stop smoking, and Mrs. White is pleased about that. She considers other things he's urged ridiculous. "What does this girl need to go to a class for having babies? She's already had two, if you remember. She knows how to do it. I never had a class and I did just fine with five kids." Miner never won out on the prenatal classes; he tried to convince Mrs. White to be the labor coach for her daughter if John wouldn't. "Coaches are for sports teams," she said. "And I have to support the family. I work." Jesse went to one class, but reported back that the teacher was "full of it" because she told the class that childbirth involved "some discomfort." "I don't know what that woman was talking about," Jesse had said. "It hurts like hell and all you have to do is go stand in one of the maternity wards when three of 'em are yelling to find that out."

Dr. Miner does an ultrasound on Jesse in the thirty-eighth week. The baby is quite large. Miner estimates that it's close to nine pounds, and he knows that if the baby goes to term before labor begins it may gain another pound or so. "You've got a nice big baby there, Jess," he says.

"Bigger than my others?"

"Let's see, how big were they, eight pounds?"

"Rosie was eight nine, and Johnny was eight four."

"Well, this one may be a little bigger than that."

Jesse smiles. "Yeah, he's been kicking like that."

"How do you know it's a he?"

"Mama can tell by the way I'm carrying. She was right for both the others."

That night Miner gets a call at home. It's Mrs. White. "Doctor, I would like you to do a cesarean section on Jesse."

"Why is that, Mrs. White?"

"You know perfectly well why. You told her yourself the baby was bigger than the others."

"Yes, it is a large baby, but Jesse's other babies were fairly large and she had no problems. I'd like to let her try to have the baby vaginally."

"Look, Doctor, don't try to pull one over on me. I know all the rich ladies get C-sections. I don't want my daughter to go through what I did with her brother Richard. I was in labor for thirty-eight hours, then they had to put the forceps on. No one should go through that. I want you to do a cesarean."

"Mrs. White, I promise you I won't let Jesse labor for thirty-eight hours. We just want to let her try. If there's a problem we'll do a cesarean."

"Why should she labor at all if that baby's going to be too big? Nine pounds already, could easily be ten."

"Lots of women deliver ten-pound babies, Mrs. White. One of my patients had one three weeks ago—her baby was over ten pounds and it only took nine hours."

"I bet if I was some rich patient, you'd play a different tune."

"I'd tell you exactly the same thing. If it had anything to do with money, Mrs. White, I'd tell all my patients to have cesareans. The hospital gets reimbursed more for them."

Mrs. White isn't convinced. She says that they'll have to discuss it further.

They don't get a chance. Two days later Jesse comes to the hospital midmorning in labor. John drove her in, but he slinks off quickly. Her mother can't leave her job but will come as soon as she's off. Jesse was completely relaxed the last two times Miner delivered her, but this time she's tense. "I'm pretty worried," she tells Miner. "Mama's sure this baby isn't going to fit."

"If he doesn't fit, we'll do a cesarean, that's all."

She looks at him dubiously. "How are you gonna do that, once he's started coming down? I won't have any choice then."

"Wrong, Jess. I can do a cesarean all right. I'll push him back up if I have to—and sometimes I do have to."

"Really?"

"Yeah, really."

A little after 5 P.M., Miner feels a tug at his sleeve as he looks over some charts at the nurses' station. It's Mrs. White. "It's been seven hours, Doctor. When are you going to stop putting my daughter through pain and suffering for no reason?"

"I checked Jess a half hour ago. She's doing great. She's eight centimeters dilated and the baby's in perfect position. There are no indications of any problems."

"You don't think pain is a problem?"

"If Jesse asks for painkillers, I'll give them to her. When I talked to her, she said she was doing fine and it felt just like the other ones."

"I don't care what she says. I am her mother and I am telling you to do a cesarean."

"Mrs. White, Jesse is nineteen. She's an adult. She makes that decision."

"She's a baby, she's no adult. I support her. She couldn't care for those babies without me. I say do a cesarean."

Dr. Miner can stick with his decision or give in to the pressure being brought by the mother. Miner knows there are plenty of doctors in his hospital who would have done a cesarean without batting an eye. A couple of obstetricians routinely do cesareans on any baby over nine pounds. Although it doesn't look as though Jesse is going to have problems, he knows things could always happen. The head could deliver, but in big babies the shoulders could get stuck, and that is a disaster.

If he speaks alone with Jesse, she'll go along with him, but if

Mrs. White talks to her, she'll change her mind. He's a bit tired of dealing with Mrs. White, but doesn't want to let that fact affect his decision.

"Mrs. White, I'll make a deal with you," Miner says. "You know as well as I that Jesse will agree with whoever she's just talked to. Let's talk to her together. I'm going to give her the choice of my doing a cesarean now or waiting till she's fully dilated and has tried pushing for an hour. If we don't have a baby by then she can go for the cesarean or keep trying—whatever she wants."

"She doesn't understand these things well enough to—"

"Then we'll explain them to her."

"All right, Doctor, but I promise you, if things go bad, if you have to use the forceps, I'll sue you."

Something that's implicit in every case, the possibility of a lawsuit, has suddenly been made very explicit. Mike Miner has been in the hospital for sixteen hours. He's tired and wishes he weren't here. Now he's got someone promising to sue him if things go wrong. He can just imagine the scene if Jesse can't deliver.

Dr. Miner turns away from Mrs. White toward the nurses' station. "OR 208. Prep the patient. I'll be scrubbed in a few minutes." He turns back to Mrs. White. "You've got your cesarean. I'll let you tell your daughter."

Forty-five minutes later he delivers a nine-pound three-ounce baby girl. Mother and infant are in excellent health. Dr. Miner doesn't see Mrs. White again; Jesse is quiet when he talks to her.

Miner goes home and tells his wife about interfering relatives and the trouble they cause. Mrs. White tells her friends how she faced down that smart-mouthed young doctor and made him do the right thing for her child. Jesse tells her friends that her mama didn't know the sex of her baby after all.

Dr. Miner's decision was understandable, but it was wrong. He did a cesarean for which he had no real medical justification. Just as important, he let down his patient. His primary duty was to Jesse and her baby. Jesse had gone along with him because she trusted what he said. She was worried—about her own well-being, about going against the wishes of her mother—but she would have trusted her doctor had he decided not to operate. Miner should have stuck with his original proposal. It was a very good idea, because it involved a strategy that allowed Jesse to participate but didn't shut her mother out of the process.

The nurses who were working with Jesse were furious with Miner for caving in. They had managed to get Jesse involved and excited. Just before the order for the cesarean had come in, Jesse had said that this labor seemed easier than the others and that she was sure her little boy was going to come out soon. She didn't say much when they started prepping her for surgery, just looked up at one of the nurses and shrugged.

Dr. Miner was tired, as he had been dealing with two other difficult cases that day as well. No one likes to be openly threatened with a lawsuit, but placating a relative is never a good basis for medical decisions.

FETAL LOSS

Pam Leuthold is a twenty-eight-year-old lawyer. She had her first child, a son, two years ago by cesarean. She has come to see Dr. Vertell Kanyama because she's heard that Kanyama is very open to letting previous cesarean patients deliver vaginally. Many of the obstetrician's patients have had successful VBACs.

In their first appointment, Pam Leuthold explains that she felt that she was pushed into the cesarean by her former doctor, an obstetrician who practices in another hospital. "I had been in labor for about sixteen hours when Dr. Mason came in and started saying stuff about dystocia. I said, 'You mean my baby's too big?' and he said, 'Yes.' Well, Jake was only seven and a half pounds. I shared a room with a woman who'd just had an eight-and-a-half-pound baby—and she'd had a cesarean before. I decided Dr. Mason must have wanted to get out to his tennis game or something that afternoon. The whole thing made me angry, and I decided I didn't want to be pushed around anymore."

Dr. Kanyama explains her philosophy: she expects previous cesarean mothers to deliver vaginally, and she has quite a high success rate—more than 75 percent of her previous cesarean patients have had VBACs. "Understand, though, that almost a quarter still end up with a cesarean. I don't make guarantees, except that you'll be given a good trial of labor and you'll participate in any decisions we make." Leuthold says she'll be back as soon as she's pregnant.

Three months later she's back, and tests confirm that she is indeed pregnant. She says that her husband, Steve, is with her all the way on the VBAC, "but the rest of my family, and his, think I'm nuts. They keep telling me to save myself the trouble. I say waking up after missing the birth of my baby, having horrible headaches, and hurting for two months is not what I call saving myself trouble."

When Kanyama sees Pam Leuthold at thirty-six weeks, her patient is a little worried. A friend who had badly wanted a VBAC had ended up with a cesarean. The friend felt like a failure, and Leuthold felt the doctor should have given her longer. She wants assurance that no one at the hospital is going to put pressure on her at the last moment. "I've got enough pressure at home."

"I'll tell you what I've told you before," Dr. Kanyama replies.

"I fully expect you to deliver vaginally. If there are problems, we'll talk about alternatives together. We'll decide what to do together."

Leuthold comes in for weekly checkups now. She looks fine at thirty-seven weeks and at thirty-eight weeks. The ultrasound shows a normal-sized baby, a little over six pounds. At thirty-nine weeks everything still looks fine. Pam is anxious to go into labor, and says she's looking forward to the delivery.

Two days later she calls Dr. Kanyama. She says she can't feel the baby moving. Kanyama tells her to come in to the hospital. "There's probably nothing wrong, but we'll take a look."

In her office, Kanyama has her patient lie down, puts a stethoscope in place, and bends over to listen. "I know it's probably nothing," Pam says, her voice nervous. "It's just that this baby's been so active. It kicks a lot harder than Jake, and I just . . ." She breaks off, watching as Dr. Kanyama continues to move the stethoscope and listen intently. The room is silent for several minutes, then Kanyama straightens up. "I'm not able to hear a heartbeat, Pam. I think we better go right in and do an ultrasound."

Twenty minutes later, Dr. Kanyama stares at the screen of the ultrasound monitor. The fuzzy image of the baby is floating there; the tiny heart is motionless. Pam is crying quietly. "I knew it," she says. "I knew it right away."

Vertell Kanyama's chest is tight. She's thinking of what her patient still has to go through. Along with her grief will be the guilt as her relatives tacitly or overtly condemn her for not being sensible and having the cesarean at thirty-nine weeks. Worst of all, the baby still must be delivered. It has died, but it hasn't disappeared. She tries to say a few words of comfort to her patient, then broaches the unavoidable topic. "I could do a cesarean, but I would recommend that you wait until you go into labor and deliver vaginally." Inwardly she's thinking, Would I want to carry and deliver a dead baby?

"Yes, that's what I'll do," says Leuthold.

Eight days later she goes into labor. The young obstetrical

nurses have never been at a delivery where the fetus was already dead. They're a little unnerved, don't quite know whether to enthusiastically urge the patient on or keep quiet. But Steve Leuthold is there and encourages his wife, coaching her as if it were a normal birth. There are moments when Kanyama can barely look at the two of them. All of the assertions she has made in VBAC classes and support sessions ring a little hollow now to the doctor.

The delivery takes just a few hours. They can find no obvious cause of the infant's death. It looks to Kanyama as if the umbilical cord may have been kinked, and she suspects that's what caused the death. She leaves the hospital more depressed than she ever has following a delivery.

Steve Leuthold calls the next day and invites her to a memorial service they're having. Vertell is grateful that the couple doesn't feel bitter. After the service she speaks with Steve. "I know another child is the last thing you're thinking about, and I don't think I should try to talk to Pam yet, but I want you to know that if you decide to try again, I'll support whatever decision she makes about what kind of delivery to choose." She also gives him the name of the leader of a support group at the hospital.

Six months later Kanyama gets a note from the Leutholds saying that the group has been helpful. A year later Pam is back in Kanyama's office. "I want to have another baby. I'm not exactly sure what I want to do about delivery. . . ."

The case has changed Kanyama's perspective. Last year, had such a patient come to her, she would have said there was no reason not to try again for a VBAC. After all, the baby didn't die because of something associated with delivery. Labor hadn't even begun. The timing of it all was just a coincidence. The baby could have died weeks earlier, when there wouldn't have been the possibility of doing the cesarean. A year ago, Dr. Kanyama wouldn't have hesitated to tell the woman that it would be foolish to risk a premature baby in order to avoid the small risk of a death of the sort that occurred. She would have said the odds of this happening again were tiny.

A year ago she hadn't gone through this, though. She doesn't want to push her patient into anything, yet she still believes in the medical soundness of VBACs. Should she take a decisive role, strongly recommend the VBAC? Announce up front that she'll be happy to do a cesarean this time? Tell the patient that it's her decision?

There's a bit of silence. Then Kanyama says, "I'm going to tell you what I told you last time. I expect you to have a vaginal birth. But I also want you to know that if you want to go to a cesarean at any time, I'll do it. If it's going to cause you too much emotional grief, it's not worth it. But if you can manage, I think we ought to do it, and I'm sure it will go well."

"I was hoping you'd say that, and dreading it a bit, too," says Leuthold. "I know the VBAC is the right thing, but I'm scared. And my whole family is against it. They told me I was wrong last time and that I'm stupid and stubborn to try a VBAC."

"I'm going to be a little scared, too, but I know we can do it."

Pam's pregnancy goes well. The last few weeks are tense. The thirty-eight-week checkup is difficult. At one point Pam asks for a date for a cesarean, but she calls back later and says she's changed her mind. The day of her thirty-ninth-week appointment she calls Dr. Kanyama. "Cancel the appointment," she says. "Meet me at the hospital. I'm in labor."

Twelve hours later, seven-pound Kelly is born.

This is one of those cases where the cesarean seems to be the "easy" choice. Certainly the death of Pam Leuthold's baby made the second VBAC decision terribly difficult. These are the kinds of cases that make it hardest for those of us arguing against unnecessary cesareans. But just because a particular decision can, in some very rare cases, lead to tragedy doesn't mean we should reject that decision. Even had Leuthold had a scheduled cesarean, the baby could have died in utero before the date. The cesarean is no guarantee against bad outcomes; it's just that in cases like these, where a cesarean scheduled in the thirty-ninth week could have saved the baby's life, it suddenly looks like the right thing to do. I maintain that it's not. If it were, then why not deliver all babies by cesarean at thirty-eight weeks? If the decision is good for the previous cesarean patient, then it's good for all. I don't think anyone will argue that we should be delivering all babies by cesarean.

THE DIABETIC PATIENT

Before the twentieth century, diabetic women very frequently died before they reached childbearing years. Those who lived often proved to be relatively infertile patients. When doctors began to understand the disease and devise ways of treating it, diabetic women became fertile, became pregnant, and became a problem for obstetricians. By the 1930s and 1940s, there was better care for diabetics, but the morbidity and mortality for both diabetic women and their infants remained quite a bit higher than the normal population. Care continued to improve, but pregnancy still caused problems. The main difficulty was that if the mother's blood sugar levels weren't controlled very well, it affected the infant. Sometimes the result was a stillborn infant. A second problem, though, was that if the mother's blood sugar wasn't controlled, her high levels reached the baby and stimulated the release of insulin in the infant. This insulin release behaved like a growth hormone, causing the baby to grow larger. The result was abnormally larger babies. Doctors often tried to counter these two problems (death before labor and large babies) by delivering the woman early by cesarean. The problem was that while early delivery avoided some problems, it resulted in another—a premature baby. Although the infants were often large for their age, they were not mature for their age. In other words, the child might already be seven pounds at seven months, the size of a normal term infant, but he or she would still only have the lungs of a seven-month-old fetus and wouldn't be able to breathe well. Until recently, doctors who delivered the babies of diabetic patients early often ended up with premature babies with all sorts of problems.

Now we have a way to find out if the baby's lungs are mature enough to enable it to survive outside the mother. Through amniocentesis we can measure the ratio of two substances in the amniotic fluid—lecithin and sphingomyelin—and determine the maturity of the infant's lungs. Thus, if the lungs are mature at thirty-eight weeks, we know we can deliver the woman without risking her baby's health. But what route should we take? There's the cesarean, of course. But diabetics are especially vulnerable to the risks of the cesarean. They tend to get infections more easily, and their ability to heal wounds is poorer than that of healthy people. What about inducing labor and delivering vaginally? Unfortunately, oxytocin, the main drug used to induce labor, doesn't work well when the woman is not close to labor. We often get nowhere if we try to stimulate a woman at thirty-eight or thirty-nine weeks if she is not ready. Oxytocin seems to be effective when the body is close to ready—it starts the contractions, and suddenly the woman's system will kick in on its own and take over. Before the woman is ready to go into labor, however, it's difficult to do much.

So some doctors routinely deliver babies of diabetic mothers at thirty-eight or thirty-nine weeks by cesarean. However, many of us are trying to take these patients to term. We've found that by rigidly controlling the woman's blood sugar levels, we can often prevent excessive growth, and if the baby is in a normal size range, there's no reason she can't deliver vaginally at term. These babies can still be fairly large, though, and managing a diabetic patient takes a great deal of attention. The decisions can be tricky.

Mrs. Irene Bailey makes an appointment with Dr. Karin Walker, an obstetrician, when she is just considering pregnancy. Mrs. Bailey is thirty-two years old, a diabetic, and otherwise in good health. She has never been pregnant and is trying to decide if she wants to try.

Dr. Walker, who is in her first year in practice, tells her that the hospital, a large urban teaching center, has a good record of delivering diabetics' babies vaginally and ending up with healthy babies. She tells Mrs. Bailey that she will have to begin a fairly inflexible regimen before pregnancy and be willing to be very conscientious about her diet and checking her blood sugar levels. "I'll want you to check them four times a day, and I don't want you to do it unless you're committed to sticking to a strict diet," she tells the patient. Bailey's records indicate that she had had some severe episodes of insulin shock during her teen years, but that she had been very good about regulating her diet since then. Once she feels confident her chances of delivering a healthy child and avoiding a cesarean are good, Mrs. Bailey decides to go ahead with the pregnancy. From the start she is very committed. She has a supportive husband who does all the cooking and eats the same things she does, so she doesn't feel deprived. Irene checks herself four times a day with her glucometer (an instrument patients use to measure their blood sugar levels).

At thirty-eight weeks, Dr. Walker orders an ultrasound. The baby is large, already about eight and a half pounds, but not yet too large to make a vaginal impossible. At thirty-nine weeks the baby is only about a half pound larger. Its lungs are mature enough to make it on their own, but both Dr. Walker and Mrs. Bailey want to wait a while and hope labor starts spontaneously.

They decide that if nothing has happened by Wednesday, which is three days before Irene's due date, she will come into the hospital and they will try to induce.

By Tuesday night nothing has happened. Dr. Walker gives Mrs. Bailey a new diet routine and tells her to come in the next day at 6 A.M. When she arrives, she's checked carefully. A nurse attaches her to the fetal heart monitor and hangs up the oxytocin to stimulate the uterus to contract. At first a drop of the drug is dripped into Irene's system each minute, then two, and finally Dr. Walker has her up to the highest dosage she will give. All day Irene is in bed. She eats nothing (she's being fed through the IV, which allows Walker to control her blood sugar level very exactly). She has occasional contractions, but is not in labor. Her cervix is not dilated at all. In the afternoon Dr. Walker tries what's called "stripping the membranes," a rather uncomfortable procedure in which the doctor tries to help induce labor by running a finger around inside the cervix and moving the bag of waters, or membrane, away from the cervix. By 5 P.M., nothing has happened, but the fetal heartbeat is very good.

This is one of those times when everyone is ready but the baby. It's difficult for both patient and doctor to wait. Although Irene isn't having any problems, her diabetes means things could get complicated. Karin Walker knows that labor could start at any time, but she also knows things could drag on for days. She's not sure she wants to put her patient through that.

The cesarean option is always there. It would be a simple thing to do. But, Walker tells herself, if there were complications, things wouldn't stay simple. And she's been working with this patient so hard to make a vaginal delivery possible. . . .

Dr. Walker decides to give Mrs. Bailey Thursday off; she hopes she'll go into labor, but if not it will give her a day of rest at home before trying induction again.

Friday morning the process starts again. Irene comes in with an empty stomach, and the nurses hang up the oxytocin. Within an hour contractions start. They look good, coming about every three to four minutes. The cervix begins to shorten a bit. But Irene's system never kicks in; the contractions aren't really labor yet. At the end of the day, the two women talk for quite a while. Irene is tired and somewhat discouraged. Finally they decide that Irene will stay in the hospital so the baby can be monitored. So far the baby seems healthy, and though over nine pounds, a vaginal birth is very feasible. If nothing has happened by Monday, Dr. Walker will try to induce again, and if that doesn't result in progress, she'll break the membrane. "Once I've done that, we'll have to go ahead and deliver, one way or another," she explains. "So you'll either be in labor getting ready to deliver Monday night, or I'll go in and do a cesarean." Mrs. Bailey agrees.

Walker sees Irene Bailey on rounds Saturday and Sunday. She's becoming more and more tense, but she's still committed to waiting till Monday. Bill, her husband, is with her as much as he can be and is supportive.

At 4:15 A.M. Monday, Dr. Walker gets a call at home. Mrs. Bailey is having contractions every two to three minutes and is three centimeters dilated. Walker rushes into the hospital, and Irene is already at five centimeters by the time she gets there.

Dr. Walker is a little nervous now. Despite the fact that many diabetics have delivered vaginally in her hospital, Karin herself has never done one (she witnessed several in medical school and residency, however). She knows the baby is still under ten pounds, but she has visions of a normal head followed by football shoulders.

By 7 A.M. Mrs. Bailey is fully dilated and has the urge to push. Second stage starts. The baby comes down slowly, and Walker can see it is fairly big—no surprise: she knew this from ultrasound. When the baby reaches S plus 3 (about one-and-a-half inches from delivery) Dr. Walker glances at the clock. It's 9:30. Mrs. Bailey has already pushed for more than two hours, and she still has a way to go. Many doctors, including some of Walker's teachers at medical school, would cut it short and go to a cesarean. If anything happens at this point—fetal problems, a difficult delivery—everyone will feel terrible. Dr. Walker trusts her instincts, though. This baby's heart has been ticking along with amazing precision, and although progress is slow, it's steady. She encourages Irene, who's also in good shape, not at all discouraged. But just to be a little safer, she has her transferred from her birthing room, where she'd rather deliver patients if she can, to the delivery room. If there's an emergency, she'll have equipment and help right on hand.

A little after 10:00 the head crowns and delivery starts taking place. After the head delivers, Dr. Walker suctions the baby's mouth and feels around, trying to see if the shoulders are going to be a problem. She can feel no cord, and she can tell this is indeed a big head, but she can't really tell anything about the shoulders. The delivery has slowed down, so she takes hold and gently pulls on the head—is there more resistance than there should be, or is it just her own nervousness? Then suddenly the anterior shoulder comes down. Now Walker knows it's all right. If that one shoulder is out she knows the baby will make it. Seconds later the posterior shoulder emerges. She pulls the baby out, and before she can even clamp the cord, the little girl is screaming. Everybody in the room laughs, Irene and her husband half crying at the same time. Kristin Bailey weighs in at 9.8 pounds, and scores a nine on her Apgar.

The best thing Mrs. Bailey and her doctor had going for them was that they could communicate well and work as a team. They both felt proud of their success in controlling the diabetes so well during pregnancy; this bound them together and created mutual trust. Irene was very discouraged toward the end. Had she not been able to draw support from Karin Walker, she might not have agreed to the last two difficult days. Similarly, Walker was able to go through the difficult process, her first, because the patient was cooperative and accepting of the frustrations they had to face.

While it is often possible for diabetics to deliver vaginally, even in difficult cases like this one, most deliver by cesarean now. Some doctors don't have the expertise to design a good program of care for a diabetic, and some are just not committed to trying to prevent the excess growth of the infant that can result in a cesarean. This should change as diabetics begin to ask for vaginal delivery and doctors no longer see an early cesarean as a good option.

THE MORBIDLY OBESE PATIENT

Mrs. Teresa Califano comes to Dr. Mark Tomsho in her eighth week of pregnancy. She has had a previous cesarean due to a diagnosis of dystocia. She went through a good trial of labor, dilated eight centimeters, then arrested there. After trying for a while, Dr. Tomsho performed a cesarean. The baby was seven and a half pounds and healthy. Mrs. Califano developed a minor infection in her incision but had no major problems. This second pregnancy appears to be normal.

Mrs. Califano is a high-risk patient, however, because she's a morbidly obese woman. She stands about five-two and weighs 280 pounds. No one likes to operate on this type of patient. It's difficult to even find the abdomen in all that flesh. Complications from anesthesia are much more common because the medication dissolves into the tissue of the fat, so the physician has to put a lot in before the needed effect is produced. Getting the endotracheal tube (the airway into the lungs) in is often difficult. Just pumping the bag to keep air in the patient is difficult because of the weight of her breasts on her chest. The lungs of such patients often do not reinflate well after surgery because there is so much chest weight pressing down on them. Finally, there is a higher incidence of blood clots in such patients. We can handle these problems, but we try to avoid any unnecessary surgery because it can so often be difficult.

Obese patients carry higher risks even for normal births. Their babies tend to be larger than average, making it more likely there will be difficulties of fit. Such patients often have what we call "soft tissue dystocia"—they're fat on the inside, too, and the tissue inside obstructs the baby. However, the risks of vaginal birth are much lower than those of cesarean for such patients.

Dr. Tomsho has suggested a trial of labor to Mrs. Califano. He feels she would benefit from avoiding an operation. She's receptive to the idea but worried about the pain. Her first labor had been difficult, and she doesn't want to go through a second painful experience. Dr. Tomsho promises he'll try to make her as comfortable as possible.

On a Tuesday afternoon Teresa Califano comes to the hospital. She's just started to have contractions. Several hours later she's five centimeters dilated and is complaining of pain. Dr. Tomsho orders an epidural. There are problems associated with the epidural: It can cause blood vessels to dilate, and the patient's blood pressure may drop. But we can compensate for this by giving the patient extra fluids and, if necessary, giving her a drug to make the vessels constrict. In addition, though, the epidural makes it impossible to move around. A normal problem in late pregnancy and delivery is that the large uterus presses on blood vessels when the woman is on her back. Blood pressure lowers and the heart has to work harder. In Mrs. Califano's case, there is not only a uterus pressing down, but perhaps a hundred pounds of fat as well. And it is difficult, and sometimes impossible, to get the epidural in the right place in the spine in these obese patients. Tomsho knows he has to be careful.

It takes Teresa ten hours to get to six centimeters. The epidural is renewed. The descent of the head is slow. Two and a half hours after full dilation, they're still struggling away. Dr. Tomsho is a little concerned about a large baby; he wishes this delivery were over with.

Five minutes later the tracings on the fetal heart monitor change. There are big U-shaped curves, indicating decelerations. It looks to Tomsho as if there is pressure on the umbilical cord.

Dr. Tomsho has to make a quick decision. He can go to a cesarean. That's the very thing he's been trying to avoid, though. A planned cesarean on this patient would have been difficult, now it will be an emergency operation. On the other hand, the baby may be in trouble. There's not much time to fool around. Yet he knows the umbilical cord compression may not be severe. The heartbeat looks good between contractions.

Tomsho has the patient moved to a delivery room and asks for the vacuum extractor. It's a device that looks something like a

FIGURE 7

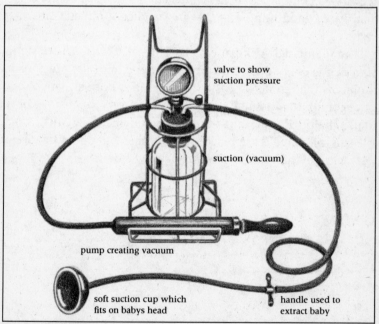

valve to show
suction pressure

suction (vacuum)

pump creating vacuum

soft suction cup which
fits on babys head

handle used to
extract baby

Vacuum Extractor

plumber's helper. It is placed on the baby's head, a pump is put through the tube, and the air is sucked out under the plastic cup, creating a vacuum. The doctor pulls a chain on the device, and it sticks tightly to the baby's head. He can then pull on the handle attached to the chain and draw the baby out.

Tomsho has the extractor on quickly. He pulls the chain and in a moment is holding an eight-and-a-half-pound baby girl. Her Apgar is seven and quickly rises to nine; she's fine, and so is her mother.

Tomsho could have done several other things when the decelerations started. He could have immediately performed a cesarean; he could have tried a forceps delivery; or he could have waited. All would have been acceptable, but none would have guaranteed a good outcome. I believe the fact that he avoided the cesarean was a good thing and that he handled a difficult situation well.

I see many high-risk patients like Mrs. Califano. The obstetrician's choices are often much more limited in these cases; many problems that could be easily handled in a normal patient can have complicated ramifications in the high-risk patient. We have to use all our clinical skills and the best judgment we can muster. We still try to avoid the cesarean if possible, but often the case is less clear-cut than cases involving healthy women.

CONCLUSION

In this book I have concentrated on the problems associated with cesarean birth. I feel that the high cesarean birth rate is cause for concern, but it's by no means an insurmountable difficulty. I am very optimistic about turning the situation around.

The first step in doing that is recognizing that what many doctors and patients have considered to be medical facts about the cesarean are in fact myths. The cesarean myths are powerful and pervasive. We doctors helped create them, and we've come to believe them, to a large extent. Women believe them, partly because they haven't been presented with the other side, partly because the myths fit so neatly with the expectations many of us have come to have: expectations of perfect results, of quick fixes, of a right to be redressed for anything that goes wrong.

The data and case studies I've presented show that the myths are not justified. The cesarean is not safer for the baby in most cases, and it almost always presents more risk for the mother—as much as four times the risk of a vaginal birth. The cesarean is not necessary in many types of cases in which it is routinely performed: the breach, the repeat cesarean, signs of irregularities in the fetal heartbeat. There are only a few types of cases in which a cesarean *must* be performed. The rest of the cases are judgment calls, situations that require the weighing of one set of risks against another. The cesarean is not "easier" for anyone, except the doctor. For the patient it means more chance of infection and other medical problems, a longer recovery, less time with her new infant, and a higher risk to her own life. Finally, the cesarean does not represent a guarantee of a good outcome. It can't save a baby who has problems that developed long before labor. Poor medical care can occur during a cesarean as well as during a normal birth. The fact that a cesarean was done does not mean that all that could be done was done.

Over the past several years I've tried to make a case against the overuse of the cesarean with my fellow obstetricians. In lectures in the National Institutes of Health report on cesarean childbirth, and in other writings I've tried to persuade my colleagues that we are not practicing good medicine when we deliver more than a quarter of babies by cesarean. I've also tried to put my message into practice, both in my own decision making during deliveries and by trying to establish, in hospitals in which I've worked, an environment in which the unnecessary cesarean is discouraged.

I decided to write *The Cesarean Myth* because I've come to realize that we can't overturn the myths without the help of patients. Further, I think patients haven't been well informed on the issue. So I hope to accomplish two goals with this book: to give patients better information on which to base their personal decisions and to enlist their help in changing the thinking and practice that have led to the rapid rise in cesarean birth rates.

To understand the development and persistence of the myths, I believe, is to go far in dispelling them. The myths grew up as the increases in cesareans were first accompanied by improvements in infant mortality and morbidity rates. The cesarean did seem to be an easy fix to a whole multitude of problems. Gradually we are realizing that it didn't fix all the problems and it created some new ones.

Once patients know that too many operations are being performed, they can best prevent an unnecessary cesarean by becoming well informed on the issue. They should understand the conditions in which a cesarean is mandatory. They should understand the conditions that may require a cesarean but often don't. They should be aware of how important the choice of a physician and a hospital are and know how to make those decisions well. They should understand that sometimes labor and delivery are long, difficult processes and be psychologically prepared. They should bear in mind, on the other hand, that although the cesarean seems "easier" at the time, the pain and difficulties are just postponed to the recovery period.

Patients should also be aware of the pressures on their doctors to do cesareans, pressures from the legal system, from their hospitals, from families of patients, and from patients themselves. They should also know about the nonmedical factors that influence the obstetrician's decision: money, convenience, and the environment in which the physician practices.

Knowing that the obstetricians may be under pressure to perform a cesarean shouldn't lead to a confrontational relationship. For one thing, I believe that *most* doctors are doing their best to make the correct decision in the complicated situations that give rise to cesarean deliveries. They often believe the myths. Even if they question them, they have to contend with the many realities associated with nonnormal deliveries, particularly the possibility of a lawsuit. For another, an adversarial relationship is usually counterproductive. One of the best ways a patient can avoid an unnecessary cesarean is to form a strong relationship with her obstetrician. A patient who understands both the complexity of the delivery room decision and the pressures on the obstetrician can begin to serve as a partner to her doctor. Unless a patient feels she's being railroaded by her doctor, confrontational tactics shouldn't be necessary. She should let her obstetrician know that she understands the issues, that she wants to try to avoid a cesarean. She should also show the doctor that she is aware of the difficulties of delivery room decisions, of the pressures, of the strength of the cesarean myths. I know that when I have such a patient, it makes it easier for me to stick with a difficult birth, to be supportive, to put aside the urge to do the "easy" thing.

Sometimes a patient may try this approach and hit a brick wall. The obstetrician will make it clear that *his* patients have no say in medical decisions, that *her* patients aren't expected to question their physician's professional judgments. Any patient who doesn't feel comfortable with her doctor or who doesn't feel she's going to be able to develop the kind of relationship she wants or to participate in the birth of her own baby should consider finding a new obstetrician. Even if the birth doesn't ultimately turn out as she expected, she'll be less likely to feel resentful or guilty over it if she had a strong relationship with her doctor.

Finally, though, I must stress that in the vast majority of cases this information won't be needed. Most people have normal labors, healthy babies, and have no medical complications. Pregnant women should be aware of possible complications, but they should also remember that the chances of them occurring are quite small. Obstetrical care in the United States is very good and has improved tremendously over the last decades. We have the highest infant survival rates per birth-weight class in the world.

We can improve care further by ending unnecessary cesareans. If good relationships can be built between doctors who reexamine their medical assumptions and approaches and patients who've educated themselves about childbirth, we can dissipate the cesarean myths. I can't say what the "correct" cesarean birth rate should be. We began to examine the issue a decade ago because we were concerned with a rate of 16 percent. Now it's 27 percent and climbing every year. Somewhere between the 4 percent rate of a few decades ago, when we were still doing too many traumatic forceps deliveries, and today's rate is a reasonable number. Clearly, 27 percent is too high. Too many women are ending up on an operating table.

Just as the situation has changed from twenty years ago, we can change it for the better. I came to Columbia University in 1985 as chief of obstetrics; in 1987 the cesarean birth rate was down 7 percent, and we expect it to continue to drop. Many obstetricians and other staff members here now assume women will deliver vaginally, and that change in attitude makes a tremendous difference in outcomes. Doctors across the country are becoming more open to VBAC and to giving women a good trial of labor before resorting to the cesarean. Patients are becoming better informed and asking for VBACs on their own. I think the outlook is good. Changes in obstetricians' attitudes are coming slowly; changes in patient attitudes could help turn the tide.

I anticipate that in the coming years the cesarean myths will be dispelled and women no longer will undergo unnecessary cesareans.

GLOSSARY

ACIDOSIS—Our bodies are in balance between the acids and the bases. When we function with less oxygen we derive our energy from other sources. This is known as anaerobic metabolism and it creates more acids, creating the condition known as acidosis. Acidosis can cause tissue damage.

ACTIVE LABOR—A woman is in active labor when the cervix is dilating. Contractions do not mean active labor.

ACTIVE PHASE OF LABOR—The period during labor when the cervix dilates more rapidly; it generally occurs when the cervix is between 4 and 10 centimeters. Contractions are stronger and more frequent.

ALBUMEN—A chemical or protein normally found in the blood. In toxemia it is often present in the urine, an abnormal condition known as albuminuria.

AMNIOCENTESIS—The process of inserting a needle in a mother's abdomen, through the skin and uterus and into the amniotic sac, to obtain amniotic fluid. Tests of the fluid can reveal information about the condition of the fetus.

AMNIOTIC SAC—The thin-walled membrane that surrounds the fetus. It is filled with a liquid called amniotic fluid that is composed primarily of fetal urine.

APGAR SCORE—This describes how alert and active the baby is after birth. Numbers are assigned for the baby's color, heart rate, breathing rate, level of activity, and muscle tone. Scores are usually taken at one and five minutes after birth. A score of 7 to 10 is normal; a good score at five minutes replaces any poor score at one minute. It was developed by

Virginia Apgar, who used it to measure how anesthetic drugs did or did not depress an infant after birth.

ARREST OF THE ACTIVE PHASE—No cervical dilations take place for at least an hour.

BREECH POSITION—The fetus is in a backside-first position, and the head, the first part to be born in normal deliveries, is the last to be born. In the frank breech, the fetus is in a cannonball position; in the full breech, a jackknife; and in the footling breech the legs and feet are the first part to be born.

CEREBRAL PALSY—A neurological disease found in children and adults. It usually involves control of muscles and movements, but may also involve intelligence. It may follow lack of oxygen, infection before birth, hemorrhage into the brain, or other conditions we have not yet identified.

CERVICAL DILATION—The gradual opening of the cervix. In pregnancy and early labor it may be closed; full dilation is 10 centimeters. Some women start labor at 2 or 3 centimeters dilation.

CERVIX—The mouth of the womb; it forms the opening of the uterus into the vagina.

CESAREAN BIRTH—The baby is extracted after the skin, underlying tissue, and uterus are incised. Also called abdominal birth.

CLASSICAL (VERTICAL) UTERINE INCISION—An up-and-down incision made in the uterus just before cesarean delivery.

CONGENITAL DEFECT—A physical defect, present before birth, indicating an abnormality from genes or chromosomes, or acquired early in the uterus. An example is a cleft lip.

CONTRACTION—The womb or uterus is all muscle tissue; it contracts to dilate the cervix and expel the uterus.

DECELERATION—When the fetal heart rate changes from a preexisting level to a lower one it is called a deceleration. Decelerations may occur following a contraction, by reflex with pressure on the fetal head, or in the presence of lack of oxygen. Most decelerations are harmless. They warrant observation because they can signal lack of oxygen.

DEHISCENCE—The separation of the skin, fat, fascia, and muscles following a surgery such as a cesarean.

DELIVERY ROOM—In the past most births took place in a formal delivery room, to which the woman was taken when her labor was almost over. Today the delivery room, with its lights and very aseptic environment, is often replaced by a "birthing room," in which the woman labors and delivers in the same bed.

DEPRESSED—The condition in which vital signs are not strong and the newborn may need assistance in starting to breathe after birth. An Apgar score lower than 6 usually indicates that the infant is depressed. The condition can be caused by lack of oxygen, too much medication, or squeezing of the umbilical cord during birth.

DIABETES—A metabolic illness of the mother in which there is either too much sugar or too little insulin.

DYSMATURITY—The fetus is either too small or not functioning as expected at its gestational age. For example, at thirty-five weeks we would expect a fetus to weigh five pounds, but the dysmature fetus might weigh only three pounds.

DYSTOCIA—Difficult labor. The term can mean that the baby was too big, the woman's pelvis was too small, the contractions were not effective, or simply that labor did not seem to be progressing normally. Because it has so many meanings, it's more useful to use more specific terms such as "arrest of labor," "failure (of the vertex) to descend," etc.

ELECTRONIC FETAL MONITOR (EFM)—This is a machine that measures the uterine contractions and the fetal heart rate at the same time, then prints them out so that the obstetrician can observe the patterns. The external monitor is one in which measurements are made by transducers placed on the mother's abdomen, while the internal monitor is one in which measurements are made by an electrode and a catheter that is placed through the vagina into the uterus.

EPIDURAL ANESTHESIA—A local anesthetic is injected to deaden the nerves coming out of the spinal column in the lower back area.

EPILEPSY—A neurologic disorder characterized by convulsions.

EXTERNAL VERSION—The process of flipping an unborn infant in the breech position into the vertex position. It is done near term and is accomplished by applying pressure to the abdomen.

FETAL DISTRESS—Clinical signs such as a falling fetal heart rate or fetal acidosis that warn that the fetus may be at risk.

FETAL SCALP BLOOD TEST—A tiny incision is made in the head of the fetus. A drop of blood is drawn up in a glass tube and analyzed to see whether the infant is experiencing acidosis.

FIRST STAGE OF LABOR—Runs from the start of cervical dilation through full dilation (it includes both the latent and active phases of labor). This is a term we try not to use today.

FORCEPS—Instruments shaped to fit around the side of the fetal head. The obstetrician slides them into place, locks them into position, and uses them to pull the fetus out.

GESTATIONAL AGE—A full term for a human fetus is forty weeks of gestation. The number of weeks from a mother's last menstrual period is the fetus's gestational age.

GLUCOMETER—A machine used to measure blood sugar.

HYDROCEPHALUS—An accumulation of spinal fluid in the brain, usually following brain damage.

HYPERTENSION—High blood pressure; it may be present in toxemia or in other maternal illnesses. Some causes of high blood pressure are not known.

INTUBATE—To insert a tube into the mouth and then beyond the vocal cords. It can be used to give oxygen or medication or to suction out unwanted substances.

IV—This literally means "intravenous." It is used to mean both the solution given intravenously and the apparatus for giving the solution.

LABOR—The process of contractions and cervical dilation leading to birth.

LABOR ROOM—The hospital room in which women labor.

LATENT LABOR—Lasts from the onset of the first contraction until the rate of cervical dilation reaches 1.2 centimeters per hour (first baby) or 1.5 centimeters per hour (subsequent babies). This slow part of labor usually ends around 4 or 5 centimeters of cervical dilation.

LECITHIN—A fetal lipid (fat) found in the amniotic fluid that comes from the fetal lung.

LECITHIN/SPHINGOMYELIN RATIO—The ratio of lecithin to sphingomyelin is related to the maturity of the fetal lungs. The ratio is determined by a test of the amniotic fluid drawn during amniocentesis and used to predict how mature the fetus is and whether the fetus will have difficulty breathing (respiratory distress) if born.

MECONIUM—Fetal bowel contents. They may be expelled when fetal distress (severe or minimal) occurs, staining the fetus and the amniotic fluid green.

MENTAL RETARDATION—Damage to the thinking part of the brain. An IQ score of 60 or less is usually considered a sign of severe mental retardation.

MORBIDITY—Medical problems or complications, such as infection, respiratory distress, or brain hemorrhage. Neonatal morbidity refers to such problems in the newborn infant. When we speak of maternal morbidity rates, we mean such problems experienced by the mother following birth.

MORTALITY—Death; maternal or fetal.

NATURAL CHILDBIRTH—A spontaneous vaginal birth, usually with minimal or no medication given.

NEONATAL—This is the newborn period. It extends from birth through twenty-eight days. The baby is called a neonate during this time, and is referred to as an infant after twenty-eight days.

OBSTRUCTED LABOR—A labor that does not progress either because of fetal size or the size of the mother's pelvis, or because of poor uterine contractions.

OXYTOCIN—A chemical produced in the posterior part of the pituitary gland that stimulates the uterus to contract. It is a material that we can manufacture; when a woman is given oxytocin to stimulate contractions, she is being given an exact duplicate of the substance produced by the body.

PERINATAL—The perinatal period extends from the twenty-eighth week of gestation through the twenty-eighth day after birth.

PERITONEUM—The very thin tissue lying under the abdominal muscle. It is cut during a cesarean.

PFANNENSTIEL INCISION—The name of the transverse incision made during a cesarean. It goes horizontally through skin, fat, and underlying muscle called the fascia. Then the muscles are separated vertically and the peritoneum is cut vertically. The next cut is made in the uterus (see transverse uterine incision, classical uterine incision).

PLACENTA—Also called the afterbirth. A part of the fertilized egg that develops as the fetus develops. The pie-shaped placenta transfers materials back and forth between mother and fetus. It also manufactures some materials for the fetus. It usually delivers after the baby is born.

PLACENTA PREVIA—The placenta normally lies in an out-of-the-way place in the uterus, but in this condition it grows over the cervix.

PREMATURE BIRTH—A fetus born at thirty-five weeks or earlier.

PREMATURE RUPTURE OF THE MEMBRANE—The amniotic membranes normally break during labor; if they break twenty-four hours or more before labor they are prematurely ruptured.

PROLAPSED UMBILICAL CORD—The umbilical cord drops alongside the fetal head (partial prolapse) or beyond the fetal head into the vagina (complete prolapse). If it is squeezed after labor starts, circulation to the fetus can be halted or interrupted.

PROLONGED LATENT PHASE—A slow labor. For women who are in their first labor, more than eighteen hours is usually considered prolonged; for others, more than twelve hours is considered prolonged.

PROTRACTION OF THE ACTIVE PHASE—A slow dilation of the cervix.

SECOND STAGE OF LABOR—Runs from full cervical dilation to birth. It is late in this stage that the "urge to push" occurs.

SPHINGOMYELIN—A fetal lipid (fat) found in the amniotic fluid that comes from the fetal lung.

SPINAL ANESTHESIA—A local anesthetic is inserted directly into the spinal canal with a needle, deadening the sensations of labor.

THIRD STAGE OF LABOR—The length of time from delivery of the infant to the passage of the placenta.

TOXEMIA—An illness that generally occurs after the twenty-fourth week of pregnancy. It involves high blood pressure and kidney and liver problems. We do not know its cause.

TRACHEA—A passageway below the vocal cords through which oxygen flows to the lungs.

TRANSVERSE—Horizontal, from side to side.

TRANSVERSE UTERINE INCISION—This is different from the incisions in the skin and fat. It is made in the uterus itself just prior to delivery.

ULTRASONOGRAPHY—A machine that uses high-frequency sound waves to tell us what is inside the uterus. It is similar to radar. The obstetrician can use ultrasound to determine fetal size, condition, and age.

UMBILICAL CORD—A soft, flexible tubelike structure that has two arteries coming from the fetus and one vein going from the placenta back to the fetus. It carries nutrients and waste between mother and unborn baby.

UTERUS—The organ within which the baby develops. It becomes quite large during pregnancy (weighing several pounds), then shrinks to almost thumb size in the nonpregnant woman.

VACUUM EXTRACTOR—A soft plastic cup attached to the top of the fetal head. A suction machine then creates negative pressure so that the obstetrician can extract the fetus.

VAGINAL BIRTH—The normal birth route in which the infant passes from the uterus, through the cervix, into the vagina, and out.

VBAC—Vaginal birth after cesarean.

VERTEX POSITION—The normal birth position of the fetus; the head is pointed down and is born first. Ninety-six percent of babies are born this way.

INDEX

abdomen:
  incisions in, 5, 19–20, 42
  pain in, 43
  preparation of, 17, 19, 39
  testing through, 16, 32
abortion, 105
abruption, 5
acidosis, 6, 33, 149, 151, 152
acquired immune deficiency syn-
    drome (AIDS), 43
adhesions, 43, 65, 66
afterbirth *see* placenta
albumin, 51, 149
albuminuria, 51, 149
alcohol, 91
American College of Obstetri-
    cians and Gynecologists, 84,
    88, 108
amniocentesis, 16, 134, 149, 153
amniotic fluid, 16, 20, 118
  fetal stool in, 33–34
  premature release of, 45, 48–
    49, 52, 117–23, 154
  substances in, 134, 152–53,
    154
  testing of, 16, 134, 149, 153
amniotic membrane, 20, 149
  infection and, 48–49, 118, 119

premature rupture of, 45, 48–
    49, 52, 117–23, 154
  rupture of, 137
  stripping of, 136
anesthesia, 15
  administration of, 3, 17–18,
    95, 139
  breathing problems and, 5, 7,
    18
  choices of, 79
  epidural, 2–3, 18, 79, 95, 140,
    151
  general, 3–4, 7, 18, 69, 70
  improvements in, ix, 16
  local, 69
  problems with, 7, 21, 64, 139
  regional, 18
  side effects of, 2, 9, 64, 70
  spinal, 2, 18, 154
anesthesiologists, 2, 4–5, 7, 17–
    18
  availability of, 42, 55
antibiotics, 21, 39, 40
antiseptic techniques, 15
Apgar, Virginia, 150
Apgar scoring system, 6–7, 69,
    96, 110, 122, 138, 142,
    149–50, 151

FOR THE BEST IN PAPERBACKS, LOOK FOR THE

In every corner of the world, on every subject under the sun, Penguin represents quality and variety—the very best in publishing today.

For complete information about books available from Penguin—including Pelicans, Puffins, Peregrines, and Penguin Classics—and how to order them, write to us at the appropriate address below. Please note that for copyright reasons the selection of books varies from country to country.

In the United Kingdom: For a complete list of books available from Penguin in the U.K., please write to *Dept E.P., Penguin Books Ltd, Harmondsworth, Middlesex, UB7 0DA.*

In the United States: For a complete list of books available from Penguin in the U.S., please write to *Dept BA, Penguin*, Box 120, Bergenfield, New Jersey 07621-0120.

In Canada: For a complete list of books available from Penguin in Canada, please write to *Penguin Books Ltd, 2801 John Street, Markham, Ontario L3R 1B4.*

In Australia: For a complete list of books available from Penguin in Australia, please write to the *Marketing Department, Penguin Books Ltd, P.O. Box 257, Ringwood, Victoria 3134.*

In New Zealand: For a complete list of books available from Penguin in New Zealand, please write to the *Marketing Department, Penguin Books (NZ) Ltd, Private Bag, Takapuna, Auckland 9.*

In India: For a complete list of books available from Penguin, please write to *Penguin Overseas Ltd, 706 Eros Apartments, 56 Nehru Place, New Delhi, 110019.*

In Holland: For a complete list of books available from Penguin in Holland, please write to *Penguin Books Nederland B.V., Postbus 195, NL-1380AD Weesp, Netherlands.*

In Germany: For a complete list of books available from Penguin, please write to *Penguin Books Ltd, Friedrichstrasse 10-12, D-6000 Frankfurt Main 1, Federal Republic of Germany.*

In Spain: For a complete list of books available from Penguin in Spain, please write to *Longman, Penguin España, Calle San Nicolas 15, E-28013 Madrid, Spain.*

In Japan: For a complete list of books available from Penguin in Japan, please write to *Longman Penguin Japan Co Ltd, Yamaguchi Building, 2-12-9 Kanda Jimbocho, Chiyoda-Ku, Tokyo 101, Japan.*